HOW TO EAT WELL AT EVERY AGE

Eating well should be easy. But so often it is not. *How to Eat Well at Every Age* provides practical tips based on psychological theory and evidence to enable people of every age to eat well and build a good relationship with food.

Eating well is key to how we interact with others, manage our emotions and our sense of wellbeing. The book describes how we can help others and ourselves to eat well across the lifespan, from good food parenting as our children are growing up, to eating well as an adult when the food environment can seem to be against us, to caring for the needs of people as they age. It describes how we learn what food we like and how our eating habits develop. It explores how parents can help their child eat well through good food parenting and the key pillars of being a good role model, saying the right things and managing their environment. It then covers how to eat well as an adult in terms of eating less to lose weight (without doing harm) or changing ingrained habits to eat more healthily in general. Finally, it explores how eating well can be key to looking after ourselves or others as they age when living independently or in residential care.

This book is for anyone who wants a healthy relationship with food, for themselves or those they care for. It is also valuable reading for students studying child development, nutrition, dietetics, catering, physical health, social care, nursing and psychology.

Jane Ogden is a Professor in Health Psychology at the University of Surrey, UK. She has published over 280 research papers and 9 books, including 4 specifically on eating behaviour. She has taught modules of eating behaviour for over 35 years to psychology, medical, nutrition, dietetic and vet students.

BPS ASK THE EXPERTS IN PSYCHOLOGY SERIES

British Psychological Society

Routledge, in partnership with the British Psychological Society (BPS), is pleased to present BPS Ask the Experts, a new popular science series that addresses key issues and answers the burning questions. Drawing on the expertise of established psychologists, every book in the series provides authoritative and straightforward guidance on pressing topics that matter to real people in their everyday lives.

All books in the BPS Ask the Experts series are written for the reader with no prior knowledge or experience. For answers to everything you ever wanted to know about issues important to you, ask the expert!

Understanding and Helping to Overcome Exam Anxiety
What Is It, Why Is It Important and Where Does It Come From?
David W. Putwain

Understanding Artificial Minds through Human Minds
The Psychology of
Artificial Intelligence
Max M. Louwerse

Rising to the Challenge of Life After Cancer
Expert Advice for
Finding Wellness
Jeffrey Charles Dunn and Suzanne Kathleen Chambers

Building a Psychologically Safe Work Environment
Binna Kandola

Understanding Climate Anxiety
Geoffrey Beattie

Living Well with Parkinson's
A Guide to a Fulfilling Life
Angeliki Bogosian

Living with Grief
A Compassionate Companion
Sara Mathews

How to Eat Well at Every Age
Jane Ogden

For more information about this series, please visit: BPS Ask The Experts in Psychology Series – Book Series – Routledge & CRC Press

HOW TO EAT WELL AT EVERY AGE

JANE OGDEN

Routledge
Taylor & Francis Group

LONDON AND NEW YORK

First published 2026
by Routledge
4 Park Square, Milton Park, Abingdon, Oxon OX14 4RN

and by Routledge
605 Third Avenue, New York, NY 10158

Routledge is an imprint of the Taylor & Francis Group, an informa business

For Product Safety Concerns and Information please contact our EU representative
GPSR@taylorandfrancis.com. Taylor & Francis Verlag GmbH, Kaufingerstraße 24,
80331 München, Germany.

British Library Cataloguing-in-Publication Data
A catalogue record for this book is available from the British Library

ISBN: 9781032987262 (hbk)
ISBN: 9781032987255 (pbk)
ISBN: 9781003600183 (ebk)

DOI: 10.4324/9781003600183

Typeset in Joanna
by Newgen Publishing UK

'I've found this book by Jane Ogden incredibly insightful. She draws on years of experience and solid research to create an easy-to-read, genuinely accessible guide to eating well—whether you're feeding a family, looking after your own health, or supporting older relatives. I loved how practical it is, with tips on what to say and do, and even some super-simple recipes that work in real life. It's a brilliant resource, especially for those of us trying to stay well in a world that often pushes us in the opposite direction'.

Kitty Dimbleby, author, journalist, communications professional, and mum of two fussy eaters

'Jane Ogden has drawn upon a wealth of evidence on psychology of food and eating behaviours, to produce an easy-to-read resource to help all of us across the lifespan live in a world that is often designed to make us unhealthy. I particularly liked the tips for eating well as we age and using food to promote wellbeing whether we are living independently or in residential care'.

Julienne Meyer, Professor Emerita of Nursing: Care for Older People

'A fascinating look at one of the most important and frequently dysfunctional relationships of our lives, with what we eat. Eating well is key to a long and healthy life so understanding why we often don't is essential!'

Mariella Frostrup

'Using her years of experience Jane Ogden has produced a very accessible guide to eating well for children, adults and in older age. Full of useful tips on what to say and do for yourself or for others – even some very easy recipes! A great resource to help us live in a world that is often designed to make us unhealthy. I will definitely recommend it to my patients as an additional tool as they learn to manage their emotional eating and for those supporting others'.

Denise Ratcliffe, Consultant Clinical Psychologist

'Jane Ogden has drawn upon years of academic experience and a wealth of scientific evidence to create an easy-to-read and accessible guide to eating well for any age. A brilliant and much-needed resource to help us all live in a world that seems to be designed to make us unhealthy'.

Alice Smellie, *writer and women's health campaigner*

'Something that affects us all daily and yet is increasingly difficult in a world designed to drive unhealthy choices and maximum profit. Jane Ogden expertly combines her many years of experience with the wealth of available evidence to produce an easy-to-read and very accessible guide to eating well for everyone; children, adults and those in their older ages alike. Full of useful tips on what to say and do for yourself or for others – even some very easy recipes! A great resource to help us live well and make choices for a healthy life'.

Lucy Jones, *Chief Clinical Officer, Oviva*

'Jane has an exceptional ability to make the complex world of health psychology engaging and deeply relevant to everyday life. This book explores how our relationships with food and eating behaviours evolve over time and the profound impact it can have on wellbeing. In a world where eating healthily can often be challenging, this book offers both transformational insights and practical tips to help support ourselves and those we care for to eat well and stay well'.

Jenna Mosimann and David Titman, *Directors of RaisingNutrition Ltd*

'People living with obesity often struggle with a food environment that makes it hard to eat well. Jane uses her many years of experience to provide a wealth of top tips and practical advice for eating well from childhood through to older age to help people look after themselves and care for those around them. All of Jane's previous books have proven to be valuable resources; I have no doubt this will be another in that series'.

Ken Clare, *Executive Director UKCPO and patient advocate*

CONTENTS

WHO AM I AND WHY AM I GIVING YOU THIS ADVICE?

Eating should be about nutrition and staying alive, and food should be a nice part of life and not a problem. But so often, it all gets far too complicated. I have seen friends always on or off a diet and endlessly criticising the way they look. I have seen some even count every calorie and watch as their weight has melted away. I have seen patients living with obesity struggle to lose weight, and when they do lose weight, they struggle to keep it off. I have heard children announce random likes and dislikes and watched as their parents desperately try to find something they will eat, and I have seen parents hover over their children pressing them to eat more, bribing them with ice cream and then wondering why they do not like vegetables. I have seen my family members age and lose weight as they forget to eat, as living alone takes all the pleasure out of cooking. And I have sat in care homes watching old people left with a plate of mush when they can hardly lift their head up. And I have also watched as the TV is increasingly dominated by chefs producing the perfect dinner whilst the viewers at home are sitting on the sofa eating ready meals.

Food is about emotional regulation, social interaction and communication. It is about identity and control. And it is about managing a food environment designed to make us overeat and eat the wrong things. This book is about eating well in a way that builds a good relationship with food and does not do harm. It explores the when, where, how and why of eating and describes how to put food back into its box. And it uses psychological theory and evidence to offer practical solutions to being a good food parent, having a good

DOI: 10.4324/9781003600183-1

relationship with food as an adult, and staying well as we age or caring for someone else as they age.

I have always been interested in the role of food in our lives. As a child, I was surrounded by diet products when everyone seemed to be 'slimming' but not losing weight. And then felt liberated when Susie Orbach announced that 'Fat is a feminist issue', which was the basis of my dissertation at university, where I argued biology was not enough to explain why we eat. I then did my PhD at London University on eating behaviour, focusing on 'The what the hell effect' and why trying to eat less can cause us to eat more.

I am now a Professor in Health Psychology where I teach psychology, nutrition, dietetics, medical and even veterinary students to think psychologically about health and hope they realise that eating behaviour is about much more than gut hormones and brain chemicals.

During my career, I have published 280 research papers to explore the mechanisms of over- and under-eating, the management of obesity as well as focusing on aspects of body image, women's health and symptom perception. I have also written nine books for both academic and lay readers.

But my passion has always been to get out of my ivory tower and bring psychology alive so that it makes sense to everyone. I teach through stories, and my students are subjected to endless anecdotes about my friends and family to illustrate research and theory. I hope this helps! I have been a consultant and on-screen expert for TV programmes such as 'Secret eaters', 'The truth about fat', 'The truth about staying slim' and 'The truth about take aways'. I also love radio and am often invited to discuss whatever the news throws up that has a psychology angle. And I write for the press and have published many opinion pieces, some of which are listed at the end of this book. I seem to have views on a lot of things these days!

So here I am, 38 years after my dissertation on eating behaviour. I know the research and theory, and have at last worked out how to turn that into advice for others. I have also listened to patients, friends and family and worked out what works for real people in their real lives, not just in the covers of academic journals. And I have brought up my own two children, now 26 and 23, and looked after my Gran for three years until she died aged 100. I am NOT a perfectionist and throughout my life and work, I have developed a very strong 'good enough' principle – I have been a good enough professor, a good enough mum, a good enough daughter and a good enough wife!

This book is about aiming high to eat well, but then being kind to yourself when standards slip and you eat 'good enough'. And it's about how to develop a good relationship with food without doing harm, so that food can be a part of life and not a problem.

INTRODUCTION

Eating well should be easy. Hunger is a basic biological drive designed to keep us well, and eating should be a straightforward and fun part of life. But so often, it is not. Our food environment is designed to make us overeat or eat the wrong foods; parents are busy, food is expensive, cooking takes time, children announce random likes and dislikes that seem to come out of nowhere, and as we age, our bodies seem to tell us to eat less, even though we need to eat more. And on top of that, people can easily develop a problematic relationship with food, where it becomes the focus of their anxiety rather than just a part of their lives.

This book describes how eating well is much more than just the nutritional content of what we put into our mouths, but reflects our relationship with food and the where, when, why and how of eating. It describes how we learn what food we like and how our eating habits develop. It explores how parents can help their child eat well through good food parenting and the key pillars of being a good role model, saying the right things and managing their environment. It then covers how to eat well as an adult in terms of eating less to lose weight (without doing harm) or changing ingrained habits to eat more healthily in general. Finally, it explores eating well as we age and how to self-care or care for others when they are living independently or in residential care.

DOI: 10.4324/9781003600183-2

Throughout, this book draws upon a range of psychological theories and evidence to answer questions such as:

How can I have a good relationship with food at any age?
How do we learn what we like?
What is good food parenting?
What should I do if my child eats too much?
What should I do if my child eats too little?
How can I help my child feel better about how they look?
Why do people diet, and what are the consequences?
How can I change my diet and lose weight?
How can I change my diet to be healthier (without making food into a problem)?
How can I have a good relationship with food?
How can I have a good relationship with my body?
How do we care for ourselves as we age?
How do we care for others living independently as they age?
How do we care for those in residential care?

WHO IS IT FOR?

This book is for anyone who wants to eat well and develop a good relationship with food. It is also for anyone who cares for others, whatever their age.

THE STRUCTURE OF THE BOOK

This book is in four sections.

Section 1 – sets the scene for the book and covers healthy eating, eating-related problems, what eating well and having a good relationship with food mean and how we learn what we like to eat.

Section 2 – focuses on children and describes good food parenting and offers solutions to problems such as not having much time to cook and having a child who will not eat a healthy diet, eats too much or too little, has poor body image and needs to be more active.

Section 3 – focuses on adulthood and addresses why people overeat, why losing weight is so hard, how people can change their diet for weight loss or just to be healthier and how adults can develop a good relationship with both food and their body size.

Section 4 – this section explores the role of food in later life in terms of both our physical health and wellbeing, and highlights how food can help with some of the changes ageing brings. It then offers some solutions for caring for others as they age, who are either living independently or in residential care.

Finally, the last chapter pulls together some of the key ideas of the book and offers some final take-home points.

A NOTE ON LANGUAGE

Mind/body interactions – I am a health psychologist who has focused on physical health for most of my career. I am aware that the division into physical and mental health is problematic, as they are clearly intertwined. But this division is a helpful tool for thinking about the role of food in our lives. I, therefore, use the physical/mental health terms throughout the book.

Person first language – Over the past decade, obesity researchers have moved to person first language, such as 'person living with obesity' rather than an obese person. There is also a debate on whether we should use the term obesity at all. This is not always the case for other diet-related conditions such as diabetes, heart disease and cancer. Throughout this book, I hope that I have used person first language where I can.

Dieting – there is a long history of dieting, and the term itself has gone in and out of fashion. To me, dieting means 'trying to eat less to lose weight'. I, therefore, use the term dieting to reflect this.

A NOTE ON DETAIL

I am an academic, and most of my writing is for academic papers and people who do research. The aim of this book is to make this research interesting and accessible to busy parents. I have, therefore, tried to include enough detail to be useful but not too much detail, which can be boring. If you want any further information, please use the recommended reading and reference lists at the end of the book.

SECTION I

SETTING THE SCENE FOR EATING WELL AT EVERY AGE

1

WHAT IS EATING WELL?

There is a huge amount written on what we should eat and what makes up a healthy diet. Eating well, however, is also about when, where, why and how we eat. This chapter will describe what constitutes a healthy diet in terms of one that is high in fruit and vegetables and complex carbohydrates and low in fat, ultra-processed food and sugary foods. It then describes the different types of food-related problems, including malnutrition, obesity, heart disease, diabetes, cancer and eating disorders. Finally, it explores how we can eat well and develop a good relationship with food at any age, focusing on the when, where, why and how we eat, the role of emotional and mindless eating and the notion of putting food back into its box.

WHAT DOES HEALTHY EATING MEAN?

A visit to any bookstore will reveal shelves of books with diets designed to improve health through weight management, salt reduction, a Mediterranean approach to eating, or the consumption of fibre. Nowadays, there is, however, a consensus among nutritionists as to what constitutes a healthy diet. Descriptions of healthy eating tend to describe food in terms of broad food groups and make recommendations as to the relative consumption of each of these

DOI: 10.4324/9781003600183-4

groups. Current recommendations for adults and children aged over 5 are as follows:

- **Fruit and vegetables**: A wide variety of fruit and vegetables should be eaten, and preferably five or more servings should be eaten per day.
- **Bread, pasta, other cereals, and potatoes**: Moderate amounts of complex carbohydrate foods should be eaten, preferably those high in fibre such as brown bread, brown pasta, and brown rice.
- **Meat, fish, and alternatives**: Moderate amounts of meat, fish, and alternatives should be eaten, and it is recommended that the low-fat varieties be chosen.
- **Milk and dairy products**: These should be eaten in moderation, and low-fat alternatives should be chosen where possible.
- **Fatty and sugary foods**: Food such as crisps, chips, sweets, and sugary drinks should be consumed infrequently and in small amounts.

Other recommendations for adults include a moderate intake of alcohol (a maximum of 3–4 units per day for men and 2–3 units per day for women), the consumption of fluoridated water where possible, a limited salt intake of 6 g per day, eating unsaturated fats from olive oil and oily fish rather than saturated fats from butter and margarine, avoiding ultra-processed foods where possible, and consuming complex carbohydrates (e.g. bread and pasta) rather than simple carbohydrates (e.g. sugar). It is also recommended that men aged between 19 and 59 consume about 2,550 calories per day and that similarly aged women consume about 1,920 calories per day, although this depends on body size and degree of physical activity.

Recommendations for children are that breast milk is best until 6 months; that up until 12 months, most nutrition will still come from milk but solids should be introduced to encourage a variety of food preferences, then until aged 2, parents should give their children a diet high in fruit and vegetables and complex carbohydrates, moderate in protein but be less restrictive for fatty foods and dairy products than for older children. By five years old, however, children should be consuming a diet similar to that recommended for adults, which is high in complex carbohydrates such as brown bread, brown pasta and brown rice, high in fruit and vegetables and relatively low in fat and sugary foods. Children should have plenty of dairy in their diet for their teeth and bones. They should also have a diet that is low in salt and should not drink any alcohol until they are at least 16. Throughout childhood, it is also important that children are exposed to lots of different types of foods; even if they announce specific dislikes, these foods are still available, and families should eat meals together as much as possible to help develop a good relationship with food.

Adults and children should also drink plenty of fluids to keep themselves hydrated. Many foods, such as fruit, vegetables, soup, and stews, are also good sources of fluid. Caffeinated drinks can make you dehydrated, but decaffeinated ones can count as part of your fluid intake.

In summary

Current recommendations for healthy eating in adults describe, a balanced and varied diet which is high in fruit and vegetables and complex carbohydrates and low in fat, ultra-processed food, and sugary foods. Children's diets should approximate this, but can be higher in fat and dairy products until the age of 5 and lower in salt. After the age of 5, children's diets should be very similar in balance to an adult's, but they still need plenty of dairy for their growing teeth and bones. But as well as making sure children eat the right kinds of foods, these early years are key to building a good relationship with food, whereby food is just part of what happens at the dinner table, where children are encouraged to try a wide range of foods. That way, food can be a part of life rather than its focus.

WHAT FOOD-RELATED PROBLEMS ARE THERE?

Healthy eating is important for children and adults in many ways. First, healthy eating in childhood helps growth and general development; second, how we eat in childhood relates to how we eat as an adult and can either protect or promote illnesses later in life; third, how we eat in adulthood can relate to physical health problems such as malnutrition, obesity, diabetes, and heart disease; finally, how and what we eat is core to mental health problems, such as Anorexia and Bulimia.

Eating to be a healthy child

Children need a healthy diet to help them develop, grow, think, and learn. Every organ that they develop, every muscle they build, and every bone they make comes from the food they eat. So, although we do not understand the exact details of how each cell in our bodies is produced, it makes sense to give children a varied and balanced diet to increase the chances that it contains what they need to grow from tiny babies into fully grown adults. Recently, there has been much emphasis on obesity and the problem of being overweight. But this is only a tiny part of the problem. Regardless of body weight or how much fat a child has, they need healthy food to grow strong teeth and bones, to make a heart that works properly, a digestive system that can do its job, a set of lungs to breathe, and a brain that can keep them alive. And this all comes from food. I remember once reading how many of the soldiers who died in the Vietnam War had heart disease, even at the age of 20, due to their diet. So, even though these men looked at the peak of their fitness due to their body size and shape, inside, they were already diseased. And if children do not have a healthy diet, some may start to feel tired and breathless, suffer from asthma or joint problems or be unable to keep up with their peers. But most will seem fine. Yet, inside, they may well be storing up problems for adulthood, as many of the problems adults face have started way before they are detected by the person themselves, let alone the health professionals they meet.

Eating well as a child for a healthy life

Understanding children's diets is important, not only in terms of the health of the child, but also in terms of health later on in life, as there is much evidence that dietary habits acquired in childhood carry on into adulthood. For example, studies show that adults prefer to eat foods that they ate as children. Long-term studies such as the Minnesota Heart Study also indicate that those who choose unhealthy foods as children continue to do so when they are older (1). There is also some evidence for the impact of childhood nutrition on adult health. For example, poor fetal and infant growth seems to be linked with problems of managing blood sugar levels at age 64, and the level of fat in the blood of the child has been shown to relate to adult heart disease. David Barker has specifically examined the role of both childhood and in utero nutrition on the development of adult illnesses and has provided evidence for his 'Fetal Origins Hypothesis'. His research indicates that early nutrition starting in the womb may relate to adult illnesses such as hypertension, heart disease, stroke, and chronic bronchitis (2).

Diet and physical health problems

An individual's health is influenced by a multitude of factors, including their genetic makeup, their behaviour, and their environment. Diet plays a central role and can contribute directly towards health. It can also impact health through an interaction with a genetic predisposition. This can result in many physical health problems, which are described below.

Malnutrition

Whilst much emphasis in Western countries is on the reduction in food intake to avoid weight gain, undereating, underweight, and malnutrition are the key problems for the developing world. Recent data from the World Health Organization (WHO) (3) concluded that 174 million children under the age of 5 in the developing world were underweight for their age, with 230 million being stunted in their growth. Further, WHO estimates that 54 per cent of childhood mortality is caused by malnutrition, particularly related to a deficit of protein and energy consumption. Such malnutrition is highest in South Asia, where it is estimated to be five times higher than in the Western hemisphere, followed by Africa, then Latin America. One common problem is the low energy content of the foods used to wean children, which can lead to growth problems and ultimate malnutrition. Breast milk is an essential source of fat for children and is often the main source of fat until the child is 2 years old. Problems occur when children are weaned onto low-fat adult food. These lowered energy diets can sustain health in the absence of illness, but are insufficient to provide 'catch-up' growth if the child is ill with infections such as diarrhoea.

Malnutrition, however, not only happens in children in developing countries; the WHO states that malnutrition occurs in virtually all countries, even when the majority of a country's population has access to sufficient food. For example, in the UK, a survey of young people aged 19 and 24 years (4) indicated that 98 per cent consumed fewer than the five portions of fruit and vegetables recommended per day (average 1.6 portions). They also consumed more saturated fat than is recommended and more sugar, mostly from fizzy drinks. Their diets were also deficient in vitamin D, vitamin A, and iron (particularly women). Likewise, adult diets have been shown to be too high in red meat, unsaturated fats, salt and sugar, and the diets of elderly people are often deficient in vitamins, too low in energy, and have poor nutrient content.

Levels of malnutrition are, therefore, common worldwide and not only a concern for developing countries. Further, whilst malnutrition may be visible due to low weight, this is not always the case, and it is common for those of higher body weights also to be malnourished, which can be missed by health professionals. Malnutrition can cause a wide range of physical problems, such as heart disease, gum disease, bone weakness, digestive issues, and kidney problems. It can also result in poor resistance to illness and make people more susceptible to infections.

Obesity

Since about 1970, adults and children have become heavier in most countries of the world. The highest rates of adult obesity are found in Tunisia, the USA, Saudi Arabia and Canada, and the lowest are found in China, Mali, Japan, Sweden and Brazil; the UK, Australia and New Zealand are all placed in the middle of the range. For children, the prevalence of overweight children worldwide has doubled or tripled in the past 20 years in the following countries: Australia, Brazil, Canada, Chile, Finland, France, Germany, Greece, Japan, the UK, and the USA. There is also literature exploring whether childhood obesity tracks into adulthood, and several studies show a link between weight in childhood and later life (5).

Obesity can cause both psychological and physical health problems. For children, living with obesity is associated with psychological problems such as low self-esteem, anxiety, low mood, and a general lack of confidence. Furthermore, they are more likely to be bullied than thinner children, which can lead to underachievement or missing school. Obesity is also associated with psychological problems in adults, such as depression, anxiety, low self-esteem, and high levels of body dissatisfaction and for some, these problems can track through from childhood right through the lifespan. Obesity is also associated with physical problems. For children, these mostly relate to being immobile and unfit and not being able to be as active as their friends and peer group, although some health problems start early, and evidence indicates that childhood obesity is associated with childhood asthma and Type 2 Diabetes. For adults, obesity is clearly associated with a wide range of physical health problems, including cardiovascular disease, heart attacks, diabetes, joint trauma, back pain, many types of cancer, hypertension, and strokes and the likelihood of these problems simply increases as a person gets heavier.

Causes of obesity

Obesity is a multi-factorial problem and illustrates a clear interplay between genetics, environment and behaviour. In terms of genetics, obesity clearly runs in families; twin and adoptee data show stronger links between those who share genes than those who share family environments only. More specifically, genetic analysis indicates that the best polygenetic risk calculation for obesity illustrates that about 8.4 per cent of body weight is predicted by genetics, which translates to about 8 kg in weight (6). Genetics, however, cannot account for the massive changes in prevalence over the past 40 years. Nor can it explain migration data, which shows how people gain weight when they move countries (7). In addition, even though our body weight is similar to that of our parents, it is even more similar to that of our friends, as it seems that body weight runs in peer groups more than it runs in biological families (8). Researchers have turned, therefore, to the 'obesogenic environment' as an explanation (9). For example, the food industry, with its food advertising, cheap ready meals, and takeaways, discourages food shopping and cooking and encourages eating out and snacking. There has also been a reduction in manual labour and an increase in the use of cars, computers and television, which makes us more sedentary at both work and home. And even if we want to be active, lifts and escalators prevent stair use, and towns are designed to make walking difficult due to the absence of streetlights and pavements and large distances between homes and places of entertainment or shops. This obesogenic environment creates a world in which it is easy to gain weight and requires effort to remain thin. I think, however, that this does not quite work as a full explanation, as although we are all living in the modern world, not everyone develops obesity. This, therefore, points to the role of behaviour – specifically physical activity and eating behaviour.

Physical activity and obesity

It is clear that recent increases in the rates of obesity coincide with people becoming less active due to all the factors in our obesogenic environment described above, such as cars, escalators, lifts, computers, television, and a desk-based society. Research also shows that being active protects against weight gain and that an inactive lifestyle can lead to overweight and obesity. Research also indicates that those living with obesity walk less on a daily basis, are more sedentary during the week and weekend, and are less likely to use stairs or walk up escalators. One study explored the relationship between body weight and floor of residence in nearly 3,000 adults across 8 European cities (10). The authors concluded that daily stair climbing may reduce weight and, therefore, should be encouraged.

Diet and obesity

Evidence for the link between obesity and diet is more complex and contradictory than for physical activity. This is in part due to problems with measuring what and how much people eat, and individual differences in how much food people need to either maintain their body weight or lose or gain weight. Further, the energy in versus energy out equation is a very fine balance, and even just eating one extra piece of toast per day, that you don't need, can result in a half stone increase in weight after a year. It is clear, therefore, that people who are overweight have eaten more than they needed in the past.

It is also clear that to maintain this level of weight, they must be eating exactly what they are using up in energy; otherwise, their weight would go down. But the details of eating behaviour and its link to obesity remain controversial. My reading of the evidence is that people with obesity may eat differently and are more likely to skip breakfast and lunch, and eat at night; they report larger portion sizes at mealtimes, show a faster initial rate of eating, and take larger spoonfuls of food (11). Further, they may be more likely to show emotional eating and use food for regulation and to manage their mood and be more likely to show mindless eating and eat because food is available rather than because they are hungry. In addition, they may be more likely to eat a diet higher in fat than carbohydrate, which may not be as effective at switching off their hunger (12,13).

Diet is, therefore, linked with obesity, which, in turn, is a risk factor for many other health problems. These problems are also directly linked to the diet itself.

Diet and coronary heart disease

The term 'coronary heart disease' (CHD) refers to a disease of the heart involving the coronary arteries, which are not functioning properly. The most important diseases are angina (chest pain), heart attack, and sudden cardiac death. Although biological factors play a part in coronary heart disease, diet is probably the fundamental factor. CHD usually involves three stages: 1) narrowing of the arteries (atherosclerosis), 2) a blood clot (thrombosis) and the impact of this, which can be sudden death, heart attack, angina, or no symptoms; this depends on 3) the state of the heart muscle. Each of these three stages is influenced by different components of the diet.

Narrowing of the arteries: The material that accumulates in the arteries, causing them to get narrower, is cholesterol ester. Cholesterol ester exists in the blood and is higher in individuals with a genetic condition called familial hypercholesterolemia. Half of the cholesterol in the blood is created by the liver, and half comes from diet. Diet influences blood levels of cholesterol in two ways. First, blood cholesterol can be raised by saturated fat found in animal fat and in boiled, plunged, or espresso coffee (not instant or filtered). Secondly, blood cholesterol levels can be reduced by polyunsaturated fats found in plant oils, soluble types of fibre, such as pectin found in fruit and vegetables, oat fibre found in vegetables, oatmeal, and oat bran, and soya protein.

A blood clot (thrombosis): A blood clot is caused by an increase in the clotting factors in the blood, including Factor VIII, fibrinogen, and platelets. Under normal healthy conditions, a blood clot is essential to stop unwanted bleeding. If there is already a degree of narrowing of the arteries, this can cause a heart attack. The formation of blood clots is influenced by diet in the following ways: a fatty meal can increase Factor VIII; smoking and obesity are associated with increased fibrinogen; alcohol is associated with decreased fibrinogen, and fish oil (found in sardines, herring, mackerel, or salmon) has been shown to help reduce platelets from clustering together and causing a clot.

The state of the heart muscle: The general healthiness of the heart muscle may determine how an individual responds to having a thrombosis. An overall healthy diet consisting of a balance between the five food groups is associated with a healthier heart muscle.

Diet and blood pressure

Raised blood pressure (essential hypertension) is one of the main risk factors for coronary heart disease and is linked with heart attacks, angina, and strokes. It is more common in older people and is related to diet in the following ways:

Salt: Salt is the component of diets best known to affect blood pressure and can cause hypertension, which is linked to heart disease, strokes, and kidney problems. As a means to reduce hypertension, it is recommended that we eat less than 6 g of salt per day, which is much less than that currently consumed by most people. Avoiding salt is difficult, however, as most of the salt consumed is not added at the table (9 per cent) or added in cooking (6 per cent) but used in the processing of food (58.7 per cent). For example, salted peanuts contain **less** salt than bread per 100 g. Many canned foods, such as baked beans and breakfast cereals, also have very high salt levels, which are masked by the sugar added. Salt is also necessary, particularly in poorer countries where diarrhoea is common, as it helps the body to rehydrate itself.

Alcohol: Alcohol consumption has several negative effects on health. For example, alcoholism increases the chance of liver cirrhosis, cancers (e.g. pancreas and liver), memory problems, and self-harm through accidents. Alcohol also increases the chances of hypertension; heavy drinkers have higher blood pressure than light drinkers and abstainers, and this has been shown to fall dramatically if their alcoholic beer is replaced by low-alcohol beer.

Micronutrients: Several components of the diet have been hypothesised to lower blood pressure, but evidence is still in the preliminary stages. For example, potassium found in foods such as potatoes, pulses, and dried fruits, calcium found in hard water, long-chain fatty acids found in fish oils, and magnesium found in foods such as bran, wholegrain cereals, and vegetables have been shown to reduce blood pressure.

Diet and cancer

Cancer is defined as an uncontrolled growth of abnormal cells, which produces tumours. There are two types of tumour: benign tumours, which do not spread throughout the body, and malignant tumours, which spread and create new tumours elsewhere (called metastasis). Diet is believed to account for more variation in the incidence of all cancers than any other factor, even smoking. But how diet affects cancer is unclear. One theory is that all foodstuffs contain natural non-nutrients which can trigger cancer. Such factors have been shown to cause mutations in the laboratory, but there is no evidence that they can do the same in human beings. A second theory claims that a poor diet weakens the body's defence mechanisms. The cancers most clearly related to diet are those of the oesophagus, stomach, and large intestine. There is also a possible link with breast cancer.

Diet and diabetes mellitus

There are two types of diabetes. Type 1 diabetes always requires insulin and is also called childhood-onset diabetes, although it can start in adulthood. Some evidence has pointed towards a role for genetic factors, and research has also indicated that it is more common in those children who were not exclusively breastfed for the first three to four months of life. Type 2 diabetes tends to develop later on in life and can often be managed by diet alone. This form of diabetes shows a clearer relationship with diet. Type 2 diabetes seems to be mainly a complication of being overweight, and the risk of developing it is greater in those who carry weight around the middle rather than on the thighs or buttocks. It is generally assumed that Type 2 diabetes is associated with diets high in sugar, as people with diabetes struggle to manage their blood sugar levels. Evidence for this association is poor, and high-fat intake seems to be its main dietary predictor, with high fibre and high carbohydrate intakes being protective.

Diet and gallstones and urinary tract stones

Gallstones are more likely to occur in women and certain ethnic groups. Obesity and dieting with rapid weight loss can increase the risk of gallstones, while moderate alcohol intake and vegetarian and high fibre diets are protective. Urinary tract stones can be made of either calcium or oxalate. Calcium stones are related to diets rich in protein, sodium, sugar, vitamin D, calcium, alcohol, curry, and spicy foods and low in cereal fibre and water. Oxalate stones are related to diets rich in foods containing oxalates, such as spinach, rhubarb, beetroot, and tea, and diets low in water.

Diet and mental health problems

Diet is, therefore, clearly related to physical health problems such as obesity, heart disease, cancer and diabetes. It is also at the core of several mental health problems. Whilst there are links between diet and a range of issues such as depression, anxiety, OCD, and addiction, this chapter will focus on eating disorders, specifically Anorexia Nervosa (AN) and Bulimia Nervosa (BN).

Anorexia Nervosa (AN)

AN is defined as involving the following factors:

- Refusal to maintain body weight at or above a minimally normal weight for age and height (e.g., weight loss leading to maintenance of body weight less than 85 per cent of that expected, or failure to make expected weight gain during a period of growth, leading to body weight less than 85 per cent of that expected). A Body Mass Index of 18 is the usual cutoff.
- Intense fear of gaining weight or becoming fat, even though underweight.
- Disturbance in the way in which body weight or shape is experienced, a central role for body weight or shape on self-evaluation, or denial of the current low body weight.
- Missing at least three consecutive menstrual cycles (for girls post-puberty or women).

There are generally two types of AN: **restricting anorexia**, which involves food restriction and no episodes of bingeing or **purging**

and binge eating anorexia, which involves both food restriction and episodes of bingeing or purging through self-induced vomiting or the misuse of laxatives, diuretics or enemas.

In the Western world, about 1 per cent of women develop AN, and although this rate increased between 1950 and the mid-1980s, it has stabilised in recent years. The majority of people with AN are female. The male-to-female ratio is 1:10, although there has been an increase in men with AN in vulnerable groups such as models, dancers, and jockeys who are required to have a lower body weight. The average age of onset is about 17 years, although there is some evidence that this is getting earlier, and some hospitals now have patients as young as 8. At such an early age, however, it is hard to see whether the child has AN or other forms of 'feeding disorder' such as 'selective eating', 'food phobias' and 'food refusal'. AN can also start in middle age or even older, and it is estimated that 1 per cent of all cases start after the age of 40, and several new cases have been recognised in women in their 70s.

All people with AN restrict their food intake. Most are extremely knowledgeable about the nutritional content of food and count every calorie. When they do eat, they tend to eat small meals predominantly made up of fruit and vegetables. They eat very slowly, sometimes cutting the food into small pieces. They avoid all fatty foods and often drink coffee and fizzy drinks, chew gum, or smoke to minimise their hunger. The diet of people with AN is often repetitive and ritualised, and they eat from a very limited repertoire. Many cook elaborate meals for others and often buy and read magazines and books containing recipes and pictures of food. Some refuse to swallow their food and chew it, and then spit it out. Others will binge on large quantities of food and then purge by using laxatives, diuretics or making themselves sick. Some also fidget when sitting, or march backwards and forwards to burn up calories. Some sufferers of anorexia also hoard food. Good descriptions of what anorexics do can be found in literature from survivors of anorexia and semi-autobiographical novels. For example, one woman said, 'I was eating fruit and dry crispbreads, lettuce and celery and a very little lean meat. My diet was unvaried. Every day had to be the same. I panicked if the shop did not have exactly the brand of crispbread I wanted, I panicked if I could not eat, ritually, at the same time' (14).

AN has very serious health consequences, and a person with AN is twice as likely to die from their condition compared to those with any other psychological problem. The most common causes of death are suicide, infection, digestive problems or heart failure caused by malnutrition. In addition, AN is damaging for teeth, bone growth and bone density, for reproductive function, and the cardiovascular system, which can cause heart problems and for the nervous system, which causes issues such as poor attention, memory loss, a poor sense of space, and slower learning.

Bulimia Nervosa (BN)

The term 'bulimia nervosa' (BN) is defined as follows:

- Recurrent episodes of binge eating. An episode of binge eating involves both 1) eating in a discrete period of time (e.g. in any two-hour period), an amount of food that is definitely larger than most people would eat in a similar period of time (taking into account time since last meal and social context in which eating occurred) and 2) a sense of lack of control over eating during the episodes (e.g. a feeling that one cannot stop eating or control what or how much one is eating).
- Recurrent use of inappropriate compensatory behaviour to avoid weight gain, e.g. self-induced vomiting, laxative use.
- A minimum average of two episodes of binge eating and two inappropriate compensatory behaviours a week for at least three months.
- Self-evaluation, overly based upon body shape and weight.
- The disturbance does not occur exclusively during episodes of anorexia nervosa.

BN can be divided into the purging type (those who binge and purge using vomiting and/or laxatives) and the non-purging type (those who binge only). The non-purging type of patients mostly use excessive exercise or dieting as a means to compensate for food intake.

About 2 per cent of women in the Western world develop BN, although this number is difficult to estimate, as many people with BN never contact the health care system. It is, therefore, about twice as common as AN. The majority of sufferers are women (male-to-female ratio is 1:10), and the average age of onset is about 18 years (slightly older than AN). Its incidence has dramatically increased since its first description in 1979, but like AN, this has stabilised in recent years.

People with BN are usually within the normal weight range and maintain this weight through the processes of bingeing and purging. Bingeing involves eating a large amount of food in a discrete amount of time; foods eaten include sweet, high-fat foods, such as ice cream, doughnuts, pudding, chocolate, biscuits and cakes. Other foods eaten include breads and pasta, cheeses, meats, and snack foods such as peanuts and crisps. Such binges are accompanied by feelings of loss of control, are usually carried out in secret, involve very quick eating, and consist mainly of the foods that the patient is attempting to avoid in order to lose weight. The consequences of a binge are described by Shute (15): 'My stomach, pressing painfully in all directions, could hold no more. I needed to collapse. Belching in rancid, vomity bursts, oozing oil from my pores, heavy and numb with self hatred … Avoiding the mirrors I pulled off my clothes, releasing an unrecognisable belly; my waistband left a vicious red stripe, but I only looked once'.

Sufferers of BN also engage in compensatory behaviour to manage any weight gain caused by the binges. The most common form is self-induced vomiting, which usually occurs at the end of a binge but also after episodes of normal eating. Vomiting is accompanied by feelings of self-disgust and loathing, is almost always secret, and may go undetected for years. Vomiting also provides a great sense of relief from the sense of distension caused by overeating and the fear of weight gain. It can become habit-forming, therefore, and encourages further overeating and further vomiting. In fact, although binge eating may start off as the primary behaviour which causes vomiting, it has been argued that over time, vomiting can start to drive bingeing. Bulimics also use laxatives and diuretics to compensate for bingeing.

Bulimia nervosa is associated with a range of physical and psychological problems. Some of these are clearly the consequences of the problem. For others, it is unclear whether they are causes, consequences, or just co-occur. Long-term follow-ups of people with bulimia indicate that about 70 per cent recover, 10 per cent stay fully symptomatic, and the remaining 20 per cent show great variability in their symptoms. The mortality rate for bulimia is much lower than for anorexia and is estimated at between 1 and 3 per cent. Those who do die appear to have received a diagnosis of anorexia at some time in their history, and the most common cause of death is suicide.

Due to nutritional deficits and the disturbance of bodily fluids caused by laxative and diuretic abuse, those with BN show cardiovascular problems such as palpitations, irregular and missed heartbeats, low blood pressure, and sometimes, heart failure. They also have digestive problems due to the movement of stomach acid and can have muscle cramps and skin problems such as dry, flaky skin, and callouses on the backs of their hands and fingers from induced vomiting. Bulimia is also associated with neurotic symptoms such as pathological guilt, worrying, poor concentration, obsessional ideas, rumination, nervous tension, hopelessness, and inefficient thinking.

In summary

What we eat is, therefore, linked to a wide range of problems. Some of these are physical health problems such as malnutrition, obesity, cardiovascular disease, cancer, and diabetes. Others are mental health problems, including eating disorders such as AN and BN. It is, therefore, key to try to eat well, not only in terms of having a healthy diet, but also in terms of developing a good relationship with food.

HOW CAN I HAVE A GOOD RELATIONSHIP WITH FOOD AT ANY AGE?

Eating well is about much more than what we eat. It is also about when, where, why, and how we eat. The rest of this book focuses on how to develop a good relationship with food and eat well at the three key stages of life: childhood, adulthood, and later life. This section will explore what a good relationship with food is (and is not) and the basic framework for achieving this at every age. In the main, I think of this as putting food back into its box!

Putting food back into its box

Food is about nutrition, reducing hunger, staying well and basic survival. Food also used to be eaten at mealtimes, tied to the dinner table, cooked in the kitchen and eaten as a family when everyone was home. But nowadays, it is also about emotional regulation, social interaction and communication and forms the basis of how we manage our moods, how we interact with our friends and families and how we see ourselves and make statements about who we are to the world around us (see Chapter 2). It is also everywhere, and we now eat at our desks, in the cinema, in the car, walking down the street and on the sofa. It has got out of its box and has taken on a much larger role in our lives than it ever did in the past. Having a good relationship with food is, in part, about putting it back in its box. It is also about allowing food to be a nice part of life, but without allowing it to become something to either worship or fear. This can be done through thinking about when, where, why and how we eat.

When and where should you eat?

Ideally, we would only eat when we were hungry, and our bodies would have an accurate notion of when this should be. For some, this is known as intuitive eating and places the emphasis on reconnecting with our bodies' biological processes. Whilst this is often promoted to enable healthy eating and reduce dieting, it relies upon the premise that we can be in touch with what our bodies need and that hunger is ultimately a physical sensation that can be detected. Much research, however, suggests that hunger is not a sensation but a perception in line with vision or other symptoms such as pain or tiredness. Therefore, in the same way that pain gets less when we are distracted from it, tiredness gets worse when we worry about it and yawning and itching can be 'caught' by watching others yawn or itch – so does hunger. These perceptions are all influenced by distraction, focus, mood and the people around us. Eating only when actually hungry is a difficult goal to achieve. 'Am I hungry – or does that cake just look nice?'; 'Am I hungry – or are we just at a café?'; 'Am I hungry – or do I just want to keep my friend company who is having a biscuit?'. If we cannot just eat when we are hungry, then when should we eat? Clearly, we should try to work out if we are hungry or not. But to make it easier, I suggest trying to pin food to specific times and places throughout the day. I have called this pinned eating, but it also fits with a vast literature on planning and goal setting, which enables people to make more considered and less spontaneous choices. So, eat at a specified time each day (breakfast/lunch/dinner), set this time ahead of the day (and ideally keep it the same each day) and try not to eat in between. Further, specify where to eat, make sure it is away from where you will be distracted (not your desk / the sofa / the car), create an 'eating space' and sit at a table somewhere and make that the place you eat. In fact, research shows that if food is called 'a meal' and eaten it sitting down 'as a meal', it might make you feel fuller than if you call it a 'snack' or eat it standing up (16). Managing where and when you eat in this way can help punctuate the day, give the day a rhythm and pass time in a nice way. It can also help you to control when (and where) you eat, make better choices and start to put food back in the box.

Why should you eat?

When a child is upset, the easiest and quickest way to calm them down is to give them food. This acts as a distraction from the feelings they are having, it gives them something to do with their hands and mouth and shifts their attention from whatever was upsetting them. If the food chosen is also seen as a treat, such as sweets or a biscuit, then they will feel 'treated' and happier. In the moment, giving food to our children to manage their feelings and behaviour is, therefore, effective. But in the longer term, it can be harmful as they are learning that food is a good way to manage their emotions. Then, as they go through life, whenever they are fed up, anxious or even just bored, they will turn to food to make themselves feel better. This is known as emotional eating and is extremely common at every age. Whilst emotional eating can help regulate emotions for many people, this often only works in the short term, as although they may briefly feel better after eating, many soon feel guilty, self-hate, and low self-esteem, which, in turn, can cause further eating. Therefore, because food is so linked with our emotions, it can lead to overeating and obesity. It can also become a core part of eating disorders as people spiral through a cycle of food and guilt. Food has, therefore, spilt out of the box and become a core part of how we manage the ups and downs of everyday life. Having a good relationship with food is about finding joy in food without that joy taking on a key role in how you regulate your life. We can eat for pleasure, but if food is allowed to become too important, it can also be quickly demonised and be allowed to damage us. Putting food back in its box is about understanding how we use food in our lives and making sure that it is to our benefit, not harm. Solutions to emotional eating involve, first of all, prevention – do not pass this on to future generations and avoid using food to manage your child's emotions! Find other ways to comfort them, such as cuddling, music, play, chat or a distraction that does not involve food. But in the present day, also first make a mental record of when and how you use food for emotional regulation and become more aware of how food works in your daily life. Then search around for other forms of self-care when your emotions need some help – keeping a diary, music, dancing, talking to a friend, fresh air, exercise, watching TV, or listening to a podcast. These will all work and will not generate feelings of guilt in the way food can do.

How should you eat?

Bags of crisps used to be 30 g, and children used to eat these and stop. Many bags are now 'grab bags' and are 60 g. Children do not eat the original 30 g, then stop and hand them back, saying, 'Mummy, I've had enough'. They eat the lot – twice the amount they used to eat. We now live in a world where portion sizes are bigger; cakes are offered around at work. We have snacks in our cupboards, and 'drive-in' fast food restaurants where we can buy thousands of calories' worth of food without even having to stop driving to eat it. And we eat it not because we are hungrier than we used to be, but because it is there. And when we are eating it, we do so without realising that we are eating, and as a result, it does not make us full. This is known as mindless eating. Research shows that if you ask someone what they ate yesterday, they will remember the food they registered as 'meals' – breakfast, lunch, and dinner. They do not remember the crisps they ate in the car on the way to work, the biscuits they had with their coffee in the morning, the cake they had in the afternoon or the burger they grabbed on the way home. And they are even less likely to remember the 'drink' they had, which had more calories hidden in it than the average meal. Recently, we did a study looking at how much people ate in four different situations: in the car, watching TV, chatting to someone, or on their own. We found two important results. First, people ate more whilst watching TV than in any of the other situations. Second, the amount they ate whilst driving was unrelated to changes in their hunger. This indicates that we eat more when we are distracted, particularly when watching TV. It also indicates that if we are so distracted, as when we are driving, we do not register the food we have eaten, and it does not make us full (17).

Such mindless eating makes people overeat in an environment where food is easily available. What we know is that most people show mindless eating. Having a good relationship with food is about mindlessly eating healthy food (eating your way through a box of grapes in the car – a good trick for children), but eating mindfully the rest of the time, so you focus on what and how much you are eating and can try and eat what you need rather than what you think you want.

Having a good relationship with food

Food is often about so much more than nutrition and involves emotional regulation, social interaction, and communication. Having a good relationship is, therefore, about putting food back into its box, allowing it to be a part of our life but not all of it! It involves managing the what, when, where, why, and how of eating so that it can be good for our physical and mental health, making it a pleasure, not a worry. It can help with our mood and sometimes even be a treat, but it should not be our main focus for emotional regulation. It can be part of how we interact with others, but not the only way, and it can be part of how we see ourselves, but not a core part of our identity. And we can eat mindlessly some of the time when the food is good for us, but try to eat mindfully most of the time, as the food environment is not always our friend. Having a good relationship with food still entails enjoying this part of our lives, but making sure that we have other ways of looking after ourselves and being with others so that food remains just a part of this, not everything.

In summary

Eating well is about much more than the nutritional content of our food. It is also about when, where, how and why we eat and developing a good relationship with food. Food can be a healthy part of our lives and a source of pleasure. But it can also become a source of guilt, self-hate and low self-esteem. Having a good relationship with food is about finding the pleasure in food without it taking over our lives, and with it still being to our benefit and not harm.

To conclude

This chapter has explored what it means to eat well. It has highlighted the role of a healthy diet and the need to eat a diet high in fruit and vegetables, moderate in protein and complex carbohydrates and low in sugary and ultra-processed foods. It has also highlighted the many physical and mental health food-related problems such as obesity, heart disease, cancer and eating disorders. It has explored what it means to eat well with a focus on where, when, why and how to eat and the role of emotional and mindless eating. Finally, it has introduced the notion of putting food back into its box as a means to develop a good relationship with food.

REFERENCES

1. Romero-Corral, A.R., Montori, V.M., Somers, V.K., Korinek, J., Thomas, R.J., Allison, T.G., and Jimenez, F.L. (2006). Association of body weight with total mortality and with cardiovascular events in coronary heart disease: A systematic review of cohort studies. *Lancet*, 368, 666–678.
2. Barker, D.J.P. (ed.). (1992). *Fetal and Infant Origins of Adult Disease.* London: BMJ Books.
3. WHO (2023). WHO guideline on the prevention and management of wasting and nutritional oedema (acute malnutrition) in infants and children under 5 years. www.who.int/publications/i/item/9789240082 830 (accessed July 01, 2025)

4. Food Standards Agency and Department of Health (2000–2001). National Diet and Nutrition Survey. Colchester: UK Data Archive. www.data-archive. ac.uk (accessed August 8, 2009).

5. Wardle, J., Brodersen, N.H., Cole, T.J., Jarvis, M.J., and Boniface, D.R. (2006). Development of adiposity in adolescence: Five year longitudinal study of an ethnically and socioeconomically diverse sample of young people in Britain. British Medical Journal, 332, 1130–1135.

6. Loos, R.J.F., and Yeo, G.S.H. (2022). The genetics of obesity: From discovery to biology. Nature Reviews Genetics, 23, 120–133. https://doi.org/10.1038/s41576-021-00414-z

7. Misra, A., and Ganda, O.P. (2007). Migration and its impact on adiposity and type 2 diabetes. Nutrition, 23(9), 696–708.

8. Christakis, N.A., and Fowler, J.H. (2007). The spread of obesity in a large social network over 32 years. The New England Journal of Medicine, 357(4), 370–379.

9. Hill, J.O., and Peters, J.C. (1998). Environmental contributions to the obesity epidemic. Science, 280(5368), 1371–1374.

10. Shenassa, E.D., Frye, M., Braubach, M., and Daskalakis, C. (2008). Routine stair climbing in place of residence and Body Mass Index: A Pan-European population based study. International Journal of Obesity, 32(3), 490–94.

11. Laessle, R.G., Lehrke, S., and Dückers, S. (2007). Laboratory eating behavior in obesity. Appetite, 49, 399–404.

12. Blundell, J.E., and Macdiarmid, J. (1997). Fat as a risk factor for over consumption: Satiation, satiety and patterns of eating. Journal of the American Dietetic Association, 97, 563–9.

13. Prentice, A.M., and Jebb, S.A. (1995). Obesity in Britain: Gluttony or sloth? British Medical Journal, 311, 437–9.

14. Lawrence, M. (1984). The Anorexic Experience. London: Women's Press.

15. Shute, J. (1992). Life-size. London: Mandarin.

16. Ogden, J., Wood, C., Payne, E., Fouracre, H., and Lammyman, F. (2018). 'Snack' versus 'meal': The impact of label and presentation on food intake. Appetite, 120, 666–672.

17. Ogden, J., Coop, N., Cousins, C., Crump, R., Field, L., Hughes, S., and Woodger, N. (2013). Distraction, the desire to eat and food intake: Towards an expanded model of mindless eating. Appetite, 62, 119–126.

2

WHY DO WE EAT
WHAT WE EAT?

We need food for survival, and when our stomachs are empty, our gut hormones and brain chemicals send signals to make us find food. But eating is about so much more than just biology. This chapter will explore the complex meanings of food with a focus on emotional regulation, conflict, social interaction, control, and communication. It will then explore how we learn what foods we like through the processes of exposure, modelling, association and control, and how our habits develop and why they are so difficult to change, emphasising repetition, reinforcement and association.

WHAT IS THE MEANING OF FOOD?

For biologists, food means staying healthy and alive. In times of famine, this is still very much the case, and we are all familiar with images of hungry children and adults in countries torn apart by war, drought, floods, earthquakes, or storms. Even in developed countries, which seem relatively stable, levels of malnutrition are surprisingly high as parents struggle to feed their children a healthy diet, or those who are homeless live from hand to mouth.

DOI: 10.4324/9781003600183-5

But fortunately for the majority in the developed world, food is not such a luxury, and because of this, our relationship with food has grown ever more wide-ranging and complex. As Todhunter said in 1973, 'food is prestige, status and wealth... an "apple for the teacher" or an expression of hospitality, friendship, affection, neighbourliness, comfort and sympathy in time of sadness or danger. It symbolises strength, athleticism, health and success. It is a means of pleasure and self-gratification and a relief from stress. It is feasts, ceremonies, rituals, special days and nostalgia for home, family and the "good old days"... a means of self-expression and a way of revolt. Most of all it is tradition, custom and security. .... There are Sunday foods and weekday foods, family foods and guest foods; foods with magical properties and health and disease foods' (1). These many meanings influence the ways in which we eat and how we provide food for those around us. In particular, food is related to emotional regulation, conflict, control, social interaction, identity, and communication.

Food and emotional regulation

In the 1970s, researchers developed the emotionality theory of eating behaviour and argued that people gained weight because they ate for emotional reasons more than thinner people. People living with obesity were, therefore, considered to eat when they were upset, bored, anxious, or for comfort, whereas those who were thinner were assumed to eat when they were hungry. Similarly, Hilda Bruch described how people with eating disorders used food to regulate their emotions and often ate because they interpreted the internal signals of emotional need as the need for food (2). Much recent research, however, indicates that most people eat for emotional reasons, not just those with obesity or eating disorders and for the majority, different foods are encoded with meanings such as comfort, pleasure, boredom, upset, and relief, and are central to celebration and the need for indulgence. And these meanings are learned from our childhood through the processes of reward and association and provide us with a rich set of beliefs about food (see the next section).

Food and conflict

Food is, therefore, strongly linked with our emotional lives and can be used as a means of emotional regulation. This process, however, generates a range of conflicts as food is often associated with opposite sets of meanings, such as eating versus denial, guilt versus pleasure, and health and pleasure.

Eating versus denial: Media images tell women, and increasingly men, that they should stay thin in order to be attractive, yet at the same time, they need to provide food for their families if they are to be a good wife and a good mother. This can create a conflict between eating and denial. As Susie Orbach stated, 'Women have occupied this dual role of feeding others while needing to deny themselves' and 'women must hold back their desires for the cakes they bake for others and satisfy themselves with a brine canned tuna salad with dietetic trimmings' (3). Food, therefore, offers a conflict, particularly for women, between eating and denial.

Guilt versus pleasure: Many foods, such as chocolate, chips, sweets, and cakes, are not only seen as a pleasure but can also generate feelings of guilt. In fact, advertising plays upon this with slogans such as 'forbidden fruit' and 'naughty but nice' and the concept of 'sins of the flesh' indicates that both eating and sex are, at once, pleasurable and guilt-ridden activities. Levine described in her book: 'I wish I were thin I wish I were fat' how 'I still feel as if I am sneaking food when I eat something I love. And I still feel guilty when I let it get the better of me' (4). These foods represent pleasure and fulfil a need. Their consumption is then followed by guilt and feelings of 'shame', feeling 'self-conscious', 'frantic' and 'perverse'.

Health versus pleasure: At times, food can also generate a conflict between health and pleasure. Parents may well be motivated to give their children a healthy diet, and the pleasure you get when they like your home-cooked healthy meal is great. BUT it is amazing how much more pleasure they sometimes seem to get from a trip to the fish and chip shop, and it is hard not to always give in to this just to get the pleasure of seeing them happy. As Marilyn Lawrence argued, 'Good nourishing food is what every mother knows her children need. She also knows that it is usually the last thing they want. Give them junk food and they will love you. But you will also have to live with the guilt about their teeth, their weight, their vitamins' (5). Food, therefore, creates a conflict between health and pleasure.

Food and self-control

Food also represents self-control, and thin people are frequently used by the media to illustrate willpower and the ability to control their desires to eat. Similarly, fasting, food refusal, and the hunger artists of the nineteenth century were and are received with a sense of wonder that they can deny themselves food. As Gordon argued, 'Hunger artists had no moral or religious agenda ... their food refusal was a sheer act of will and self-control for its own sake' (6). Further, Hilda Bruch, a psychotherapist, described the anorexic as having an 'aura of special power and super-human discipline' (2). Not eating food, therefore, means willpower and self-control. In contrast, however, overeating and being overweight are often used by the media to represent a lack of willpower and an inability to stand up to the powerful drives to indulge. Food is, therefore, related to issues of control, with some showing strict control, but the majority showing both control and episodes when this control is lost.

Food and social interaction

Food is also central to the ways in which we interact with others. We have special meals for 'The birthday party' and 'Sunday lunch', and festivals such as Christmas, Thanksgiving, Easter, Passover, Hanukkah, Diwali, and Ramadan all involve food and sometimes fasting, which is ended with a celebratory meal. Food is also a common tool for connecting within the family, and the dinner table is often the only place where the family get together to share their experiences of the day. We also eat differently with others than when we are alone, and there are many implicit rules about eating in company, such as eating a similar amount, at a similar speed and the same number of courses as others around us. That's why we often ask 'who's having a starter?' or 'who's having a pudding?' when we eat out, as to eat alone whilst others watch would feel strange and uncomfortable. In particular, food can be a symbol of family love, of power within families or society, of sexual attraction, and of religious identity.

Food as family love: Providing a meal for the family is one of the most basic ways to express love and caring, and putting time and effort into food preparation makes this love and caring seem more apparent. Similarly, eating food that has been carefully prepared by others is also the most basic way to accept this love and show yours in return. Therefore, the simple daily exchange, 'Dinner's on the table!' followed by, 'Thanks, Mum, that looks lovely!' is a central part of how families show their love for each other. And that is why, when children say, 'Err! What's that? I don't like potatoes', deep down, they know they are going to have a strong effect! Food signifies love, and disrupting this is guaranteed to make an impact.

Power dynamics in the family: For many centuries, men have been given larger amounts of food than women, children, or the elderly, and if meat is scarce, men will often be given it over the other family members. Some men are also served first, and when food is running low, the woman may well give herself the scraps so that the others can remain well-nourished. Food can also, therefore, reflect power dynamics within a family. Even in the modern family where equality is assumed, watch who gets the 'best bits' of meat or the crunchiest roast potatoes. Quite often, this indicates where the power balance lies.

Food as social power: Food is also a symbol of social power and social status. Up until about the 1920s, all powerful men were portrayed as portly to signify that they had enough to eat and were in a powerful position in society. In contrast, the poor were thin with the look of the 'consumptive' as they had less money and therefore less power. Nowadays, however, in the Western world, those in powerful positions are often thin and are portrayed as such by the media. This is not to suggest that they do not have access to food, BUT that they do have access but have chosen not to eat much of it. Denial and food avoidance have, therefore, come to symbolise having power over the social world. For example, when political prisoners need to make a social statement, they refuse to eat and initiate a hunger strike. Similarly, the suffragettes in the early twentieth century also turned to hunger strikes as a political protest over gender inequalities.

Food and sexuality: Some foods are also linked with sex and sexuality. Advertisements for ice cream offer their product as the path to sexual fulfilment; chocolate is often consumed in an erotic fashion, and the best-selling book 'The Joy of Sex' by Alex Comfort was named after the 'Joy of Cooking' and was subtitled 'A gourmet guide to love making'. This relationship between food and sex is central to many cultures and many times. Rites of passage ceremonies depicting the onset of sexuality involve practices, such as washing with the blood of a goat, killing the first animal and eating red meat, which are often considered to arouse sexual drives. History tells us that a captain of a slave ship stopped eating meat to prevent him from lusting after female slaves. Similarly, low-meat diets were recommended in the nineteenth and twentieth centuries to discourage masturbation in young males. At a more prosaic level, 'going out for dinner', 'a dinner for two' and 'a candle lit dinner' are frequent precursors to sex.

Food as religious identity: Food is also embedded with meanings associated with religion and religious identity. Many religions, such as Islam, Judaism, and Hinduism, involve rules on which foods can and cannot be eaten and the ways in which foods can be combined. In addition, religious ceremonies and festivals are recognised through food preparation and food sharing, whether it is the Turkey at Christmas, chocolate eggs at Easter for Christians, or feasts on Holy days such as the end of Ramadan. Therefore, eating food, preparing food, and providing food for others becomes a medium through which holiness can be communicated within the family and a sign of religious identity and religiosity.

Food as self-identity and communication

Food has many meanings in terms of emotional regulation, conflict, control, and social interaction. Central to all these meanings is food as a vehicle for communication. Food can be used to make statements such as, 'Who am I?', 'How am I feeling?', 'What do I feel about you?', and 'How do you make me feel?' People can use food to make statements about their emotions ('I am fed up', 'I am bored'), about how they feel about other people ('I love you', 'I appreciate you'), and about how others make them feel ('You make me feel sexy', 'You make me feel loved'). They can also use food to communicate that things are going wrong ('I am unhappy', 'I feel unloved', 'I need to be looked after'). And because food is used in this way, we quickly learn to 'read' what someone is saying through the way they eat. So, when we see someone refusing to eat, we know they are saying, 'I am unhappy'; when they cook us a lovely meal, we know they mean, 'I care about you', and when they buy us a box of chocolates, we read this as, 'You are special'.

In summary

In times of hardship and famine, food means health and staying alive. But for those where food is freely available, the meanings of food have become wide-ranging as food takes on an increasingly complex role in our lives. Food is linked with emotional regulation as people eat to manage stress, or when they are bored or fed up. It also generates conflicts between eating, denial, guilt, and pleasure. Furthermore, food is embedded with issues of control and is central to the ways in which we interact with others. Finally, food is often a way to make statements about who we are, how we feel about others, and how they make us feel. For the majority, these meanings are part and parcel of the daily process of choosing which foods we like, which ones we are going to eat, and how we are going to feed others. For the minority, however, these complex meanings of food can result in eating becoming a more destructive and damaging form of behaviour.

HOW DO WE LEARN TO LIKE THE FOOD WE LIKE?

When asked why and when they eat, most people say, 'I like it', 'It tastes nice', 'I was hungry', and 'I couldn't eat anymore'. Such explanations are in line with a more biological model of eating behaviour, which suggests that food choices are governed by innate taste preferences and the biological sensations of hunger and fullness. But people eat differently according to their culture, ethnicity, and family history. When they move from one country to another, their diets and food preferences change, and when people share their lives with others from different backgrounds, they adjust their food choices accordingly. Given the enormous cultural diversity in food preferences, it is generally accepted that food choice is more complex than simply a matter of innate preferences or biological drives. To reflect this perspective, psychological models of eating have been developed, and they focus on how we learn to like the foods we like from the moment we are born (and possibly even before), and how our preferences are shaped by the people around us, with a focus on exposure, learning from role models, learning by association and parental control.

Exposure

The theory of exposure simply describes the impact of familiarity on food preferences. Human beings need to consume a variety of foods to have a balanced diet, and yet show fear and avoidance of new foods (called neophobia). Young children will therefore show neophobic responses to a new food, but must come to accept and eat foods which may originally appear to be threatening. In line with this, studies show that simply exposing children to foods over and over again can change their preferences. In fact, several studies indicate that the magic number is about 10 times. So children in the UK like pizza, Chinese children like rice, and Japanese children like fish, NOT because their taste buds are different, but because this is the food they are familiar with. And if a British child were transported to Japan, very soon they would like Japanese food and vice versa. If we want someone to like different food, we need to keep giving it to them.

Learning from role models

Modelling describes the impact of watching other people's behaviour on our own behaviour and is sometimes referred to as 'social learning' or 'observational learning'. Early research by Albert Bandura focused on aggression and showed that children became more aggressive if they had watched an adult being aggressive. Eating is no different, and much evidence shows that we learn what foods we like from a number of role models, including peers, parents, and the media.

One early study explored the impact of 'social suggestion' on children's eating behaviours and arranged to have children observe a series of role models eating foods different to what they were used to. The role models chosen were other children, an unknown adult, and a fictional hero. The results showed a greater change in the child's food preference if the model was an older child, a friend or the fictional hero. The unknown adult had no impact on food preferences (7). In one study, children who liked peas (but not carrots) were sat next to children who liked carrots (but not peas) at lunch for a week. By the end of the study, the children had changed their vegetable preference and were eating both peas and carrots. This was also found several weeks later when the children were followed up (8). Therefore, simply watching other children changed the foods that children liked and ate. In another study, children with a history of being a picky eater watched a video with older children called 'food dudes' enthusiastically eating a wide range of foods and making comments such as 'these beans are so crunchy'. The results showed that after exposure to the 'food dudes', the picky eaters changed their food preferences and started to eat fruit and vegetables (9). Food preferences change through watching others eat.

Parental attitudes to food and eating behaviours are also central to the process of modelling. For example, we know that parents and their children of all ages tend to like and eat the same foods. We also know that even when children leave home, they tend to eat in a similar way to their parents in terms of snacking, what they eat at mealtimes and even how much they eat. In fact, even if children break away from their parents' diets in their teenage years, they tend to return to them after their rebellious period is over and they start to settle down (10). So, parents are an important source of learning and often the best way to change a child's diet is to change the parents' diet first.

Television, social media, and films are also ever-increasing sources of role models, and although cigarette and alcohol advertising has been banned in most Western countries, food advertising has not. One study analysed the nutritional content of food on television aimed at children under 5 years and showed that unhealthy foods were given almost twice as much airtime as healthy foods (11). Another study evaluated the impact of exposure to food-related adverts (12). Children with different body weights had their snack food intake measured after viewing a series of food and non-food-related adverts. The results showed that all children ate more after exposure to the food adverts than to the non-food adverts. Similarly, researchers (13) showed children adverts for healthy or less healthy foods and found that they could remember more of the less healthy than the healthy foods. Likewise, one study (14) reported that partic-ipants ate more food if they had watched a movie clip where a char-acter continued to eat rather than had finished eating. Likewise, given the recent expansion of food media in terms of food magazines, food blogs, and food adverts, research suggests that food marketing has a direct effect on eating behaviour, with children eating more food when they have been previously exposed to it (15).

Learning by association

The third psychological mechanism that influences how we learn to like foods is learning through association. The classic early study was by Ivan Pavlov, who showed that if he rang a bell each time he gave his dog some food, after a while the dog started to sali-vate when the bell was rung, even if the food was not there. Pavlov argued that the dog had learned to associate the bell with food and, therefore, reacted in the same way to the bell as he reacted to food. This is known as 'conditioning'. Similarly, Skinner showed that if he rewarded pigeons for pressing a lever with food, then they learned to press the lever more often. This is known as 'reinforcement'. In terms of eating behaviour, there is a wealth of research showing that both conditioning and reinforcement help us learn which foods we like; we like foods if we associate them with positive feelings or situations AND if we are positively reinforced for eating them. There are three ways that learning changes what we like to eat:

Rewarding healthy eating: If you say to a child, '**If you eat your vegetables, I will be pleased with you**', and then smile and praise them when they do, after a while, they will start to actually prefer these foods. The foods become associated with praise; praise is nice, so the foods become nice. Rewarding eating behaviour seems to improve food preferences. Similarly, if you give your child broccoli and pull a face saying, 'Try it, but you might not like it; it's a strange taste', they will associate broccoli with something unpleasant and will not grow to like it.

Using food as a reward for good behaviour: If you say to a child, '**If you are well behaved, you can have a biscuit**', you are using food as a reward to change a child's behaviour. This has positive effects on their behaviour in the short term and makes it more likely that they will do their homework, go to bed on time or tidy their room. BUT in the longer term, studies show that using food as the reward makes them see the biscuit as special and a treat, and therefore, makes them like it even more. So, using food as the reward is a useful short-term trick to get children to behave as we want them to, but in the longer term, it promotes a preference for unhealthy 'treat' foods. THEN, in the future, when they are feeling fed up, bored or lonely, these treat foods are the perfect solution, as this is what they have been taught as a child. This can be the root cause of emotional eating as an adult.

Using food as a reward for healthy eating: Many parents say, '**If you eat your vegetables, you can eat your pudding**', and use unhealthy food as a reward for eating healthy food. This, again, may work in the short term, and children will eat their vegetables. But in the longer term, they are learning that pudding is a treat and that vegetables are not nice, as 'my mum has to bribe me to eat them'.

In an early study, researchers told children stories about imaginary foods called 'hupe' and 'hule' and said, 'There were two foods on the table, but Jenny could only eat the "hupe" if she had eaten the "hule"'. The children listening were then asked which one they would like to eat the most, and they all wanted the 'hule' – the reward one! (16). Rewarding food with food may work in the short term, but in the longer term, it teaches the child to prefer the treat food as this is being framed as special and something that needs to be earned.

We, therefore, learn to like the foods we like through learning by association and reinforcement. If we reward healthy eating through smiling and praise, then this seems to work and can help children to prefer a healthier diet. But if we use unhealthy foods to reward either good behaviour or healthy eating, then although this may be a useful quick fix, in the longer term, children will learn to prefer the foods that have been offered as treats and avoid those foods that we really want them to eat.

Parental control

The next factor that seems to impact how we learn to like certain foods is the role of parental control. We currently live in a world where crisp bags are getting bigger; burgers and chips are offered as a mid-afternoon snack, and sweets and chocolate are sold at child height just when you are frantically sorting out your shopping trolley, and resistance is low. Many parents, therefore, impose some form of control over what their child eats. Birch (17) reviewed the evidence for the impact of imposing any form of parental control over food intake and argued that it is not only the use of foods as rewards that can have a negative effect on children's food preferences but also attempts to limit a child's access to foods. She concluded from her review that 'child feeding strategies that restrict children's access to snack foods actually make the restricted foods more attractive'

(17). For example, when food is made freely available, children will choose more of the restricted than the unrestricted foods, particularly when the mother is not present (18,19). From this perspective, parental control would seem to have a detrimental impact on a child's eating behaviour. In contrast, however, some studies suggest that parental control may reduce weight and improve eating behaviour. For example, Wardle et al. (20) suggested that 'lack of control of food intake [rather than higher control] might contribute to the emergence of differences in weight'. Similarly, we also found that greater parental control was associated with higher intakes of healthy snack foods (21). Following this research, I carried out a series of studies exploring the possible costs and benefits of parental control and argued that these conflicting results are due to parental control being more complex than acknowledged by existing measures. In particular, I examined the impact of differentiating between 'overt control', which can be detected by the child (e.g. being firm about how much your child should eat) and 'covert control', which cannot be detected by the child (e.g. not buying unhealthy foods and bringing them into the house) (22). The results showed that these different forms of control differently predicted snack food intake and that, while higher covert control was related to decreased intake of unhealthy snacks, higher overt control predicted an increased intake of healthy snacks. Similar results were also found in another sample of parents with small children (23), indicating that while some forms of control may well be detrimental to a child's diet, others may be beneficial. Further, in a longitudinal study, Jarman and colleagues (24) reported that increased covert control by parents over a 2-year period predicted healthier children's diets by follow-up, whereas an increase in overt control was associated with increased neophobia. It would therefore seem that controlling the child's environment in terms of what food is brought into the house, or which cafes and restaurants they visit, may encourage healthy eating without having the rebound effect of more obvious forms of control to overeat.

There is a consistent problem, however, with much of the research exploring parental control; it uses cross-sectional designs, which limit conclusions about causality. For example, it may well be that increased parental control causes a child to eat more. But it may also be that parents use more parental control because their child already overeats. To address this problem, I carried out two experimental studies to explore the impact of imposing parental control versus no control on a child's eating behaviour (25). We chose two naturally occurring times when children are bought chocolate: Easter eggs and chocolate coins at Christmas. For both studies, parents were randomly allocated to either the control condition (limit the chocolate to set times and amounts) or the no control condition (allow the child to have whatever they like) and rated their child's preoccupation with the target food and other sweet foods at the start and end of the interventions. The results showed that children ate less chocolate in the control conditions. But by the end of both interventions, children who had had their intake controlled showed greater preoccupation with the food that had been controlled. This study provides experimental evidence for the causal link between parental control and a child's food intake. But it could not differentiate between covert and overt control, as all parents needed to allow the chocolate into the house for the study to take place. How to use control in a helpful way with children is described in Chapters 3–5, with adults is described in Chapters 6–8, and with the elderly is described in Chapters 9 and 10.

In summary

Although we may believe that we eat because we like it or when we are hungry, eating behaviour and food preferences are much more complicated than some innate drive to keep us alive. Eating is a cultural and psychological behaviour that is learned from the moment we are born and is influenced by simple exposure and familiarity, learning from role models, by association, and in response to the ways food is controlled by our parents. How to help children develop healthy habits and deal with issues of over- or undereating and poor body image is covered in Chapters 3–5. How to help ourselves as adults is covered in Chapters 6–8, and how to help ourselves and others as we age is covered in Chapters 9 and 10.

HOW DO OUR EATING HABITS DEVELOP AND CHANGE?

Have you ever tried to give up smoking, exercise more, drink less, stop saying peculiar little phrases that slip out without thinking or change your hairstyle, or the kinds of clothes you wear? We are creatures of habit who generally like our routines and rituals and feel safest in our comfort zones. Eating behaviour is no different, and most of the ways we eat and the foods we like have been learned from an early age and involve a minimal amount of thought and effort. They feel almost instinctual. And that is how habits feel – almost instinctual. So, we clean our teeth every morning without planning to and because if we did not, it would feel wrong. We put our deodorant on often without even knowing we have done so, and we choose our breakfast without any hesitation. So, how do habits develop and why are habits so hard to change?

How do habits develop?

It is Monday morning. The alarm clock goes off, and you drag yourself out of bed. You make your way downstairs and, with half-closed eyes, flick the kettle on, put the tea bag in your favourite mug, put two pieces of toast in the toaster and get the Marmite out. Well, that is what I do and have been doing since I was about 14! You might have a shower first, you might have cereal, porridge, or muesli, or a boiled egg. And if you are Japanese, you might have rice, or a strong espresso and a pastry if you are Italian. But most of us will do this with very little thought or conscious decision-making. On a Saturday morning, we might think, 'What shall I have today?' but on a Monday, we use the smallest amount of thought and processing capacity as possible. And then we find that we are dressed, have cleaned our teeth, and are nagging the children to speed up without quite knowing where the morning has gone or how this has all happened. These are habits, and they require very little thinking and have been bedded down over many years of doing the same thing over and over again. Most of what we eat, how we eat, and how much we eat is also a habit, and has become ingrained from a very early age.

Habits are formed through three very simple processes: repetition, reinforcement, and association. When we repeat a behaviour several times, it quickly becomes a pattern. It then becomes a habit if it is reinforced by something positive, such as we like it, someone else likes us doing it, and it makes us feel good. This is even true for 'bad habits' as these also make us feel good at some level or another. Then it becomes a strong habit if it becomes associated with something in our environment or our inner mood. Take teeth cleaning. We clean our teeth every morning because, as children, our mum nagged us to do it. After a while, this repetitive behaviour becomes a pattern. Then it becomes a habit because we like it, it makes our breath feel fresher, forgetting to do it makes us uncomfortable, and sometimes people tell us, 'Your breath smells'. Finally, we then learn to associate cleaning our teeth with walking past the bathroom, the sound of someone else cleaning theirs, the smell of toothpaste or the last task to do before coming back downstairs in the morning. We have a habit, and not doing it leaves us with a sense that something is not quite right. And this feeling that something is not right is just uncomfortable enough for us to want to keep carrying on with our habit.

For breakfast, it is the same pattern. Lots of people do not like breakfast as they are 'too tired', 'it makes me feel sick' or 'I just can't eat in the morning'. This is because their normal behaviour is not to eat, and eating feels strange. But then get them to eat breakfast every morning for a couple of weeks, and soon a new pattern will be set (repetition). They will start to like the feeling of being more alert and

spending a few minutes each morning sitting quietly eating (reinforcement), and this new behaviour will be triggered by seeing the
fridge, smelling someone else's toast, or simply getting out of bed
(association). Then, not eating breakfast will start to feel strange as
their new normal behaviour has been established.

These habits, whether they be teeth cleaning or eating, are all
established from a very early age and become so entrenched in our
daily lives and the things we say about ourselves that they require
very little thought or effort to do, but a lot of effort to change.

Why are habits difficult to change?

Habits are difficult to change as, ultimately, in the moment of doing
any behaviour, its benefits outweigh the costs. So, although smoking
might cause lung cancer, at the moment of having a cigarette, the
immediate feeling of stress leaving your body far outweighs the risks
of dying in 20 years. Similarly, eating cake may add to your weight
problem, but at the time of eating cake, the pleasure of its taste and
texture cancels out the fear of having a heart attack when you are
60. Habits are, therefore, the result of a simple cost/benefit analysis,
and mostly, we are hopeless at thinking about the future, so that the
immediate benefits pretty much always outweigh the future costs.
This process is facilitated by a number of different factors as follows:

Triggers: Because habits have been created by associating the behaviour with a number of triggers, either in the environment (the
fridge) or our mood (feeling fed up), they are difficult to break, as
every time we come across this trigger, we are prompted to behave in
a particular way. And because habits require so little thought, much
of the time we are not even aware of what we are doing. So, smok-
ers get off the train and light up, if leaving the train is their trigger,
and those who overeat, eat biscuits with their afternoon cup of tea,
as this feels normal and not doing so does not feel quite right. Such
environmental triggers, however, can be avoided if we make small

changes to our daily routines or change our environment. But it is the internal mood triggers that are more difficult to manage, as they follow us everywhere and are hard to ignore.

Worry and stress: Habits are part and parcel of our everyday normal lives, and, therefore, when we do not clean our teeth, eat breakfast, have our morning coffee, or have biscuits in the afternoon, we feel unsettled and a little bit stressed. This feeling is unpleasant, and we quickly learn that it can be avoided by carrying on with our habit. Therefore, stopping smoking makes people feel stressed. This stress goes away once they have a cigarette. Similarly, not eating biscuits feels unusual, but this can all be made OK with a few biscuits. And the habit carries on as it becomes the solution to the problem created when trying to change it! It is a vicious circle. But children do not smoke, and do not find this difficult, and they feel fine when they do not clean their teeth or eat breakfast. So, it's the change in the habit which makes us feel stressed, NOT the absence of the actual behaviour. And if we start to realise that the feeling of stress or worry is just 'withdrawal' and will only be made worse in the longer term if we give in and use the habit to get rid of it, then we can start to break the habit itself.

Scripts in our heads: From an early age, we develop scripts in our heads of what we like and don't like, who we are and what we do. These scripts come from the people around us, particularly our parents, and tell us whether we are good or bad people. For example, some people have negative scripts in their heads which say, 'I am always late', 'I'm a problem', 'I'm selfish', 'I never try my best', or 'I'm stupid'. Other people may have more positive scripts which tell them, 'I am kind', 'I am thoughtful', 'I work hard', 'I always stick at things', and 'I'm clever'. In terms of habits, these scripts can make it very difficult to change if we tell ourselves, 'I am addicted to smoking', 'I have a problem with food', 'cigarettes are the only way I can relax', 'eating is my only crutch in life', or 'I have an addictive personality'. Although some of these scripts may feel 'true' and reflect how people actually behave, they make it more difficult to change, as breaking a long-standing habit not only means changing the behaviour but also changing the very way in which a person sees themselves. And this is hard.

Social pressure: We live in a social world and spend much of our time with other people. Our behaviours are, therefore, intricately linked with other people and are often central to the ways in which we build up our relationships. So, we may have a friend at work who we go outside and smoke with, a colleague who we have cake with in the afternoon, a husband who likes to buy us chocolates as a treat, or children who we enjoy taking out for ice cream. If we then try to change our behaviour, these other people in our lives may well object, and the pressure is on to behave the way we always have done. Husbands will feel rejected if we do not eat the chocolates; our friend will feel lonely smoking on their own, and we will miss out on the gossip; ice cream will seem less of a treat. People like us to carry on the way we always have, as it makes them feel safe. If we change, then they feel that they have to change, and that is unsettling. The social pressure always increases to maintain the status quo whenever anyone tries to break a habit. I remember a woman, once, who was part of my research and was trying to lose weight. Her rather unpleasant husband wanted her to lose weight and used to say, 'Here comes the elephant' when she got ready for bed. She went on a diet and was doing really well. Then suddenly he started to buy her chocolates! We have recently been exploring the impact of negative social support and identified the role of being a feeder, saboteur, and colluder (26–30). Whilst often meant as a sign of love, our social worlds can undermine our attempts to be healthier. But it is not always that well-intentioned!

Denial: When people try to change their habits, they are mostly attempting to stop doing something they still want to do. So those stopping smoking, still like smoking but know they should not smoke, people on a diet like chips but try not to eat them, and those trying to be active would rather be on the sofa but try to drag themselves off to an aerobics class. This makes changing behaviour difficult because it always introduces an element of denial, and human beings are hopeless at denying themselves something if they want it and it is available. Furthermore, the process of denial makes the behaviour we are trying to deny ourselves even more attractive and desirable than it was before. So, if we say to ourselves, 'Today I will not eat cake', automatically, we think about cake more, not less. Then, because we are thinking about cake more, but cannot have it, we want it more as the day progresses. Eventually, when we give in and have cake, not only do we now want it more than we did in the morning, but we end up eating more cake because we have been denying ourselves all day. This is a very powerful effect, which means that by making food forbidden and putting ourselves into denial, we paradoxically become more preoccupied, and when we do give in (which most people do), we paradoxically eat more than if we had not denied ourselves in the first place.

In summary

Habits are formed through the simple process of repetition, reinforcement and association and can become almost automatic and without thought as we go about our everyday lives. They are also very difficult to change because they have often been entrenched for a very long time. They illustrate a simple cost-benefit analysis, and at the time of carrying out the behaviour, the immediate benefits will always outweigh the longer-term costs. In addition, changing habits is made even more difficult due to environmental triggers, the stress and worry generated when we try to change, social pressure from others who want us to carry on as usual and the problem of denial.

In conclusion

The answer to the question: 'Why do we eat what we eat?' is far more complicated than just biology. Food has many meanings and is linked with our emotions, issues of control, how we interact with others and our identity and how we see ourselves. We learn to like certain foods through the simple processes of exposure, modelling, reinforcement, and association, which start the moment we are born (and possibly before) as our eating behaviour is shaped by the world we live in and the people we encounter. As a result, we develop likes and dislikes and use food to fit into our daily lives. We also develop habits that can often feel automatic and can be very hard to change. This is the basis of our relationship with food and can be tracked through from childhood across the lifespan. But these preferences and patterns can be changed. The rest of this book addresses how to set up a good relationship from the outset with our children and how best to develop it in adulthood and later life.

REFERENCES

1. Todhunter, E.N. (1973). Food habits, food faddism and nutrition. In M. Rechcigl (ed.), Food, Nutrition and Health:World Review of Nutrition and Dietetics, 16. Basel: Karger, 186–317.
2. Bruch, H. (1985). Four decades of eating disorders. In D.M. Garner and P.E. Garfinkel (eds.), Handbook of Psychotherapy for Anorexia Nervosa and Bulimia. New York: Guilford Press.
3. Orbach, S. (1978). Fat is a Feminist Issue ... How to Lose Weight Permanently – without Dieting. London: Arrow Books.
4. Levine, M.J. (1997). I Wish I Were Thin I Wish I Were Fat. New York: Fireside.
5. Lawrence, M. (1984). The Anorexic Experience. London: Women's Press.
6. Gordon, R.A. (2000). Eating Disorders: Anatomy of a Social Epidemic, 2nd ed. Oxford: Blackwell.
7. Duncker, K. (1938). Experimental modification of children's food preferences through social suggestion. Journal of Abnormal Social Psychology, 33, 489–507.
8. Birch, L.L. (1980). Effects of peer models' food choices and eating behaviors on preschoolers' food preferences. Child Development, 51, 489–496.

9. Lowe, C.F., Dowey, A., and Horne, P. (1998). Changing what children eat. In A. Murcott (ed.), *The Nation's Diet: The Social Science of Food Choice*. London: Longman, 57–80.

10. Dickens, E., and Ogden, J. (2014). The role of parental control and modelling in predicting a child's relationship with food after they leave home: a prospective study. *Appetite, 76*; 23–29.

11. Radnitz, C., Byrne, S., Goldman, R., Sparks, M., Gantshar, M., and Tung, K. (2009). Food cues in children's television programs. *Appetite, 52*(1), 230–233. https://doi.org/10.1016/j.appet.2008.07.006

12. Halford, J.C., Gillespie, J., Brown, V., Pontin, E.E., and Dovey, T.M. (2004). Effect of television advertisements for foods on food consumption in children. *Appetite, 42*(2), 221–225. https://doi.org/10.1016/j.appet.2003.11.006

13. King, L., and Hill, A.J. (2008). Magazine adverts for healthy and less healthy foods: Effects on recall but not hunger or food choice by pre-adolescent children. *Appetite, 51*(1), 194–197. https://doi.org/10.1016/j.appet.2008.02.016

14. Zhou, S., Shapiro, M.A., and Wansink, B. (2017). The audience eats more if a movie character keeps eating: An unconscious mechanism for media influence on eating behaviors. *Appetite, 108*, 407–415. https://doi.org/10.1016/j.appet.2016.10.028

15. Livingstone, S. (2007). Do the media harm children?: Reflections on new approaches to an old problem. *Journal of Children and Media, 1*(1), 5–14. doi:10.1080/17482790601005009

16. Lepper, M., Sagotsky, G., Dafoe, J.L., and Greene, D. (1982). Consequences of superfluous social constraints: Effects on young children's social inferences and subsequent intrinsic interest. *Journal of Personality and Social Psychology, 42*, 51–65.

17. Birch, L.L. (1999). Development of food preferences. *Annual Review of Nutrition, 19*, 41–62.

18. Fisher, J.O., and Birch, L.L. (1999). Restricting access to a palatable food affects children's behavioral response, food selection and intake. *American Journal of Clinical Nutrition, 69*, 1264–1272.

19. Fisher, J.O., Birch, L.L., Smiciklas-Wright, H., and Piocciano, M.F. (2000). Breastfeeding through the first year predicts maternal control in feeding and subsequent toddler energy intakes. *Journal of the American Dietician Association, 100*, 641–646.

20. Wardle, J., Guthrie, C. A., Sanderson, S., and Rapoport, L. (2001). Development of the children's eating behaviour questionnaire. *Journal of Child Psychology and Psychiatry, 42*, 963–970.

21. Brown, R., and Ogden, J. (2004). Children's eating attitudes and behaviour: A study of the modelling and control theories of parental influence. *Health Education Research: Theory and Practice, 19*, 261–271.

22. Ogden, J., Reynolds, R., and Smith, A. (2006). Expanding the concept of parental control: A role for overt and covert control in children's snacking behaviour. *Appetite, 47*, 100–106.

23. Brown, K., Ogden, J., Gibson, L., and Vogele, C. (2008). The role of parental control practices in explaining children's diet and BMI. *Appetite, 50*, 252–259.

24. Jarman., M., Ogden, J., Inskip, H., Lawrence, W., Baird, J., Cooper, C., Robinson, S., and Barker, M. (2015). How do mothers control their preschool children's eating habits and does this change as children grow older? A longitudinal analysis. *Appetite, 95*, 466–474.

25. Ogden, J., Cordey, P., Cutler, L., and Thomas, H. (2013). Parental restriction and Children's diets: The chocolate coin and easter egg experiments. *Appetite, 61*, 36–44.

26. Ogden, J., Cheung, B., and Stewart, S.J.F. (2020). A new measurement tool to assess the deliberate overfeeding of others: The feeder questionnaire. *Clinical Obesity, 10*(4), e12366. doi:10.1111/cob.12366. Epub 2020 May 3.

27. Ogden, J., Cheung, D., and Hudson, J. (2022). Assessing feeder motivations and behaviour within couples using the Feeder Questionnaire. *Appetite, 179*. https://doi.org/10.1016/j.appet.2022.106285

28. Ogden, J., and Quirke-McFarlane, S. (2023). Sabotage, collusion and being a feeder: Towards a new model of negative social support and its impact on weight management. *Current Obesity Reports, 12*, 183–190. https://doi.org/10.1007/s13679-023-00504-5

29. Quirke-McFarlane, S., and Ogden, J. (2024). Care or sabotage? A reflexive thematic analysis of perceived partner support throughout the bariatric surgery journey" *British Journal of Health Psychology, 29*, 835–854. doi:10.1111/bjhp.12733

30. Quirke-McFarlane, S., and Ogden, J. (2024). Is anyone else's husband trying to undermine them all the time?: A reflexive thematic analysis of online support forum discussions about bariatric surgery saboteurs. *Journal of Health Psychology.* doi:10.1177/13591053241305946

SECTION II

CHILDHOOD – GIVING YOUR CHILD THE BEST START

3

HOW CAN I BE A GOOD
FOOD PARENT?

Feeding children should be easy. Hunger is a basic biological drive, and eating should be a straightforward and fun part of family life. But so often, it is not. Parents are busy, food is expensive, and cooking takes time; even when you have managed to prepare the family meal, children announce random likes and dislikes that seem to come out of nowhere. And on top of all that, we have the fears of obesity and eating disorders looming in the background. How do we get our children to eat healthily when they do not like healthy food? How do we get them to eat more without making them overweight? How do we keep them at a normal weight without giving them an eating disorder? How do we get them to be more active when all they want to do is watch TV or play on their phone? And what do we do about a daughter who starts to obsess about her weight? This chapter will cover what good food parenting is with a focus on being a good role model, saying the right things and managing their environment. It will then provide some useful tips for how to cook healthy food when time is short and how to encourage a child to eat a healthy diet.

DOI: 10.4324/9781003600183-7

WHAT IS GOOD FOOD PARENTING?

Many children and adults develop problems with food, which can ruin their lives, whether it is because they are too fat or too thin, feel too fat or too thin, or just find food difficult. Being a good food parent involves making sure your child develops a good relationship with food, not only in terms of what they eat, but also when, where, how and why they eat. We learn our eating habits through the basic psychological processes of exposure, modelling, reinforcement and association. Being a good food parent, therefore, involves the three key pillars of being a good role model, saying the right things and managing their environment (1). I have pulled these together with examples in Figure 3.1.

As parents, we are in charge. We may not always feel like it, but we have the money, the car, and do the shopping and cooking; although we get pestered, bribed, or even bullied to do it their way, we are still in charge, at least for a while. So, if you are a good role model for how you eat and feel about the way you look, make your home a healthy home, and say the right things about being active, eating, body size and shape, then you have done your best to set your

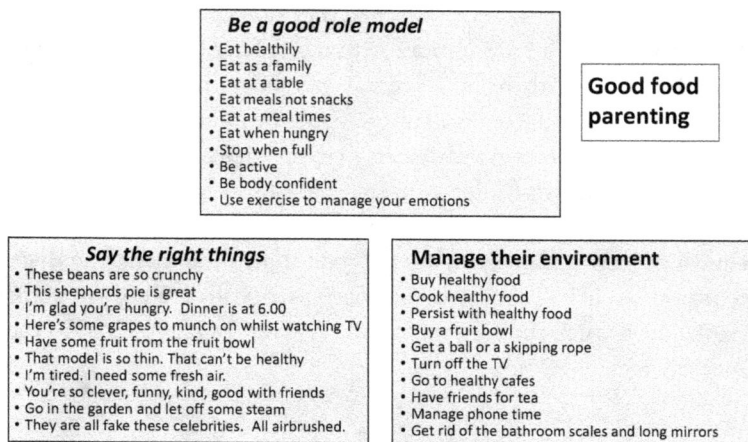

Be a good role model
- Eat healthily
- Eat as a family
- Eat at a table
- Eat meals not snacks
- Eat at meal times
- Eat when hungry
- Stop when full
- Be active
- Be body confident
- Use exercise to manage your emotions

Good food parenting

Say the right things
- These beans are so crunchy
- This shepherds pie is great
- I'm glad you're hungry. Dinner is at 6.00
- Here's some grapes to munch on whilst watching TV
- Have some fruit from the fruit bowl
- That model is so thin. That can't be healthy
- I'm tired. I need some fresh air.
- You're so clever, funny, kind, good with friends
- Go in the garden and let off some steam
- They are all fake these celebrities. All airbrushed.

Manage their environment
- Buy healthy food
- Cook healthy food
- Persist with healthy food
- Buy a fruit bowl
- Get a ball or a skipping rope
- Turn off the TV
- Go to healthy cafes
- Have friends for tea
- Manage phone time
- Get rid of the bathroom scales and long mirrors

Figure 3.1 Good food parenting.

child up for the world outside. Hopefully, although they may rebel at points along the way, as they grow up, you will have given them a solid start in life that will stay with them forever.

Be a good role model: Be a good role model and be seen to eat the foods you want them to eat. So, eat at the table with them, eat the food you want them to eat, and talk about them in a way that will make them want to eat them. Try not to snack and if you do eat healthier snacks and if you do have any problems with food, try to keep these to yourself rather than share and possibly encourage them in your children. Also, be a good role model for being active and doing exercise and how you feel about your body size. Evidence shows that parental modelling has a powerful influence on what children eat, as well as their body image and how they feel about themselves.

Manage their environment: By far the best way to control what a child eats is to manage their environment without them even knowing it. So do not bring foods into the house that you do not want them to eat, but take them to healthy cafes and restaurants and cook them food that is good for them. This way, you can have some say in what they eat, but you will not make them preoccupied with what they cannot eat. Also, set a daily structure. We live in a world where we tend to have three meals spread across the day. Children, therefore, have to learn this pattern in order to fit in. This also means that they need to learn that feeling hungry before a meal is a good thing, as food is on its way, and they will enjoy their meal more the hungrier they are. It is therefore fine to limit your child's snacking and say, 'Please don't have any more biscuits, I'm cooking dinner. You can have them afterwards'. Finally, also set a meal structure. We want children to eat more savoury, unsweetened foods than puddings, so they also need to learn that any puddings come after the main meal. This way, they will use up their hunger on the healthy foods and feel less hungry by the time dessert arrives. It is, therefore, also fine to say,

'Please wait now and have a biscuit after dinner'. BUT do not make the biscuits the reward for eating dinner; they just come afterwards!

Say the right things: Part of being a good role model and managing the environment is also choosing how you talk about food. The words we use are all part of how children embed food with meaning, and this will, in turn, change how they eat as they go through their lives. Speak positively about healthy food, and when you are around healthy food, speak about it in ways that make your child think they are nice. Say, 'This shepherd's pie is great', 'This cauliflower is really crunchy', or 'These carrots are so sweet'. And soon they will learn to eat what you are eating without any idea that they are learning these things because you want them to. Praise in the form of words and smiles can also change what they eat, so when they try broccoli and say they do not like it, say, 'Well done for trying. It was quite nice, really'; when they eat all their sausages and mash, say 'Well done – you did enjoy that!' When they say they cannot eat anymore as they are full, say, 'That's fine. It's good to know when you have had enough'. Using words in the right way can encourage a positive relationship with food. It can also be key to making sure children eat more without using too much pressure. Young children, in particular, get bored with sitting at the table and often want to get down after the first few mouthfuls. It is fine to say, 'Just eat a bit more', or 'Stay at the table a bit longer' or 'Just a few more vegetables'. But the line between encouragement and pressure is a thin one, so try to do this in a light-hearted manner, and if they really do not want to eat anymore, then leave them alone. Too much pressure will make them rebel and ultimately associate food with feeling uncomfortable. Using the right words can also help children eat less without setting up rebound effects or making them preoccupied with the wrong foods. For example, saying, 'Don't have that biscuit now as dinner is at 6. Have it after if you are still hungry' is far better than saying, 'Here's a massive easter egg, but you can't have any until the weekend'. Tying sweet food to after dinner gives it a time and a place in the day without making it a reward for eating the main meal. In contrast, buying sweet foods and then banning them can make them extra special and set up craving and preoccupation. In later life, these meanings of food then guide what we turn to when we are unhappy and how we try to manage our emotions when we need a boost.

The role of parental control

The impact of being a good role model, managing the environment, and saying the right things all illustrate the key role of parental control and how this can impact what children eat. Chapter 2 explored the different types of control and the ways they can change a child's eating behaviour. In essence, there are helpful and unhelpful ways to control what your child eats.

Helpful control: The goal of helpful control is to have some say in what your child eats, so that you can encourage them to have a healthy diet, without making them preoccupied with the very foods you want them to avoid, AND without giving them something to rebel against later on. If you make healthy eating into an obsession, once they hit their teens and really want to annoy you, they will use food as the perfect tool. But if you do it without them realising it, you give them nothing to rebel against when the time comes. So if you are a good role model and eat the foods you want them to eat in front of them, create a healthy home with structured mealtimes and healthy food and use your words carefully around food you can impose some element of control without doing harm, without making them preoccupied with the foods you do not want them to eat and without giving them something to react against later on.

Unhelpful control: Most other forms of control can be unhelpful and may do harm. And although they might offer an immediate quick fix, in the longer term, a child may well learn to prefer the foods you are trying to get them to avoid. In fact, many studies show that as they grow up, children tend to prefer the foods that have been banned, and when their parents leave the room, they reach straight for the foods that have usually been restricted. Unhelpful forms of control also take the form of what you do and what you say, and can backfire as the child grows up. Here are different forms of unhelpful control and descriptions of what children are learning when they are used:

Overt restriction: If you bring unhealthy food into the house that you would rather your child not eat, then you will need to control their behaviour in ways that they will know about. This is known as 'overt control' and might involve having a sweet cupboard that they cannot reach, a chocolate drawer that is for 'mummy and daddy' or 'special occasions', or a huge cake that they can only have a small slice of. So, try not to say, 'Those are mum's biscuits. Not for you. You can't have any', 'Just have a small piece of cake now. Have some more tomorrow', or: 'That's enough Easter egg now. Save the rest for later'. Imagine your partner buying you the perfect necklace (ring, boots, perfume, cake?), then placing it in a glass jar and not letting you have it! Pretty soon, you would be cross and obsessing about it, AND sneaking down in the night to smash the jar into pieces. This may well be what some children feel like when they know you have bought something that they are simply not allowed to have, as they learn that these foods are special and forbidden, which is a toxic combination.

Rewarding food with food: As described in Chapter 2, rewarding food with food can backfire in the longer term and is a form of control which does not really work. So, try not to say: 'Just five more peas please, then you can have some ice cream' or 'Eat your vegetables, then you can have pudding'. They might eat their five peas, but will have learned that ice cream and pudding are much nicer.

Pressure to eat between meals: When my children were little, I observed many mums giving their children food even when their child did not seem hungry. So, they would say, 'How about another slice of cake?' even when the child had not asked for it or 'You look tired. Have a piece of chocolate to give you some energy'. If children are pressured to eat even when they are not hungry, they struggle to learn what hunger feels like and then fail to learn that eating takes that hunger away. Children need to get hungry between meals so that they learn to manage this sensation, and as adults know, this sensation means 'get ready to eat soon' rather than 'I am unhappy or bored or lonely'. Anticipating your child's every need may feel like attentive parenting, but it prevents a child from learning what their own needs are and how they can fulfil them on their own.

Pressure to eat at meals: I have also observed many mums hovering around their child at teatime, spooning in extra food (way after the child could feed themselves), and going beyond the usual encouragement that is sometimes necessary. I was brought up by war children for parents who had experienced rationing and real hunger, and was often told, 'Please clean your plate. Plenty of people would be glad of that food', or 'If I could, I'd send that to the poor starving children in Africa'. Wasted food was a real sin, and we were encouraged to eat everything in front of us. Nowadays, children are subjected to other forms of pressure, such as, 'That took me ages to cook. Please eat it all', and 'Do you know how much that cost?' None of these are very helpful approaches as the child learns to eat according to what is there rather than how hungry they are. And this, again, means that they do not learn to recognise the feeling of hunger and that eating will make it go away. Sometimes, parents also get their children to eat the food they would like to eat themselves but cannot because they are on a diet, saying, 'Those chips are lovely. Do finish them off', or 'Eat that last biscuit for me, will you'. So the child eats when they do not want to, and the parent uses them as a human dustbin!

I have summarised helpful and unhelpful things to say to children in Table 3.1.

Table 3.1 Helpful and Unhelpful Things to Say to Children

Helpful things to say	Unhelpful things to AVOID saying
This shepherd's pie is great!	I know broccoli isn't very nice, but it's good for you.
This cucumber is really juicy!	
These carrots are so sweet!	Have something healthy for a change.
Well done for trying. It was quite nice, really!	After tea, we can have something nice.
Well done – you did enjoy that!	Those are mum's biscuits. Not for you. You can't have any.
You are so good at trying new foods.	
You are good at knowing when to stop eating.	You do have a huge appetite
It's good to know when you have had enough.	You are a bottomless pit!
Just eat a bit more	She does really like her pudding!
She's so good at eating vegetables.	He has a really sweet tooth!
Stay at the table a bit longer.	Just have a small piece of cake now. Have some more tomorrow.
Just a few more vegetables.	
Please don't have any more biscuits; I'm cooking dinner. You can have them afterwards.	That's enough Easter eggs now. Save the rest for later
We have a lovely melon for pudding	No, you can't have pudding. Not until you have eaten your meal.
Please wait now and have a biscuit after dinner.	
If you are hungry, have some fruit	Just five more peas, please, then you can have some ice cream.
Dinner is at 6. Just wait now.	
Here are some lovely carrot sticks to munch on before bed.	Eat your vegetables, then you can have pudding
	You look tired. Have a piece of chocolate to give you some energy.
	That took me ages to cook. Please eat it all.
	Eat that last biscuit for me, will you?

In summary

Giving a child a good start in life means trying to be a good food parent so you can help your child develop a good relationship with food. The three key pillars of good food parenting are being a good role model, managing their environment and saying the right things. These three strategies enable you to encourage eating well without creating many food-related problems in later life. This approach also involves the use of helpful rather than unhelpful aspects of parental control as trying to control what your child eats through too much pressure, using food as a reward or saying the wrong things can cause rebound effects whereby your child will react against what you say and want to do the opposite once they start to take control over what, when and how they eat.

HOW CAN I COOK HEALTHY FOOD WITH LITTLE TIME?

On my shelf, at home, are several cookery books designed for mums with endless recipes for pasta dishes, pizzas, casseroles, or sandwiches presented as hedgehogs, cats, clowns, and smiley faces. They are all unused with no evidence of splashed food anywhere! Mums are busy people. Many work as well as having children, and those who stay at home are busy managing the home and seeing to the children. Time is precious. Here are some of my own rules of thumb for making your child's diet as healthy as possible and keeping your own sanity. At the end of this book are a number of recipes that my friends and I have put together that have kept our families eating healthily and us sane.

Cook whenever you can

Home-cooked food is pretty much always healthier than eating out or eating takeaways, so try to cook as often as you can. Processed foods, pre-prepared foods, takeaways and TV dinners may be labelled as 'low fat', 'healthy eating', 'low calorie', or 'low sugar', but the chances are they are higher in all these ingredients than the food you can cook at home. I do not like cooking, I never watch cookery programmes, and I find cooking a chore. But fortunately, children seem happier with simple, easy-to-prepare, quick-to-prepare and non-fussy meals, to elaborate meals described by the latest 'family-friendly' chef. So, if you are busy, do not want to or do not have the time to prepare several courses, then STILL cook, but cook simple meals that do not take time but are still healthier than anything you could eat out or bring in.

Finding time

I had a rule of thumb that I would spend no more than 30 minutes every weekday getting food prepared from fridge (or freezer) to table. On two days a week, I spent only 20 minutes all in, as my kids had clubs to get to. Most ready meals take at least 15 minutes to reheat, and takeaways take time to order in, collect, or wait for them to be delivered. I have, therefore, become very efficient at working out how to cook quick meals that are still healthy. They may not be particularly exciting and certainly would not make it on any TV show, but they are good enough. So, set a time each day for dinner, work out how much time you have to prepare something, remind yourself that home cooking is pretty much always better than what you can buy in, and start chopping.

Buy ingredients, not meals

When you shop, buy ingredients rather than meals, and that way, you will pretty much always have something in the house to cook. Basic ingredients that I think every weekly shop should include are:

For your cupboard: potatoes, brown bread, brown pasta and brown rice, tinned tomatoes, several jars of pesto, and baked beans.

For your fridge: cheese, bacon, sausages (meat or veggie), ham, cucumber, red peppers, carrots, onions, and tomatoes.

For your freezer: chicken breasts, frozen peas, beans, broccoli and cauliflower, minced lamb or beef, meatballs, fish fingers.

These ingredients will then provide you with many possible meals that can keep you going through the week. AND they will keep you going much longer than if you buy ready meals or processed foods.

Shop for the week

Whether you shop online or go out, try to shop for the whole week rather than just a few days. That way, you will not run out of food to cook and will be able to keep going for longer. Also, try to share the workload with your partner. If you do the cooking, then get them to do the shopping. It can be done at any time throughout the week, including weekends and evenings, and if you are not convinced that they will buy the right things, give them a detailed list until they get the hang of it. If you are on your own, then this is more difficult, but try shopping online and make sure you still buy plenty of ingredients rather than meals to make it all last longer.

Make life easy for yourself

Healthy food does not have to be complicated or time-consuming to prepare. In fact, it is often the unhealthiest foods that take the most effort. So, make life easy for yourself by preparing simple meals. There is nothing wrong with foods such as sausages, mash and peas, pasta and pesto sauce, pasta and bacon and cheese, OR chicken and rice and beans. And fish fingers and oven chips, baked beans on toast, jacket potatoes and cheese, and beans are all fine. Just make sure that you add vegetables, such as chopped cucumber, peppers, carrots, or tomatoes on the side, and your family will have a quick, healthy meal, and you will have kept your sanity.

Prepare food in advance

Freezers are great inventions. When you have time, bulk cook shepherd's pie, fish pie or just bolognaise sauce. Or when you are cooking the evening meal, simply double the quantity to have next week. Then, when preparation time is short, get it out of the freezer in the morning, and the evening meal can be quickly reheated when you get back. In fact, most ovens now have a timer on so you can set it all up to go when you leave in the morning.

Roll meals over from one day to the next

As part of my efficiency drive, I have discovered the art of rolling one meal over to the next. So, if one day, we are having sausages and mash, I cook twice the amount of mash, and the next day, we have shepherd's pie or fish pie as the mash is already made. If we are having spaghetti bolognese, I cook twice the amount of bolognese sauce, freeze it and have lasagna or chilli a few days later. I also cook extra boiled potatoes so the next day, we can have them fried, and if we have a roast at the weekend, I keep the meat to go with rice on Monday. If you are weaning babies, then leftover vegetables are great for them to munch on. Older children might get bored with food if you serve the same meal on two consecutive days, but if you serve the same food but disguised as another meal, they do not notice.

Having 'help yourself' meals

Some days, I run out of steam and feel so bored with cooking. Then we have 'help yourself' meals. This involves putting bread, butter, cucumber, chopped carrots, tomatoes, ham, peppers, cheese, hummus, and any old leftovers from the fridge on the table and asking everyone to help themselves. The kids see it as a real picnic treat, and it is about as efficient as you can get.

Cutting corners

There are some things that I do that some people would be horrified by, but they make my life easier.

- I never peel potatoes, but chop them up as they are, and we are all used to eating mash with the skin in it.

- I rarely peel carrots, but just wash them first.
- I never peel mushrooms.
- I microwave meat to defrost it even though it says not to.
- I put pans on the table for serving rather than putting food in bowls
- We eat a lot of frozen vegetables with everything.

Eat as a family at a table (if you can)

Family meals have been shown to be helpful in so many ways. They encourage children who are not keen on eating to eat more, and they discourage those who would overeat. They also enable children to see food as a social event that is done at a table at set times of the day, which prevents snacking, grazing, and mindless eating. And they offer a time when everyone can take time to stop their busy lives and chat about the day. In addition, as a parent, you can use the family meal as a time to be a good role model for your child and be seen to try new foods, enjoy healthy foods, and get pleasure from seeing them eat healthily. Whilst you are preparing the dinner, get the children to set the table. This can save you time and get them involved in the cooking process.

Give yourself days off

Seven days a week is a lot to fill with healthy meals, and can become a real chore and a source of resentment if you are not careful. So give yourself some days off. Takeaways or ready meals are not great as they are mostly full of salt and preservatives. But now and then, they do no harm. So, when you have had enough, reheat a pizza, call in a curry, or have fish and chips. But try to add a salad on the side or reheat some frozen peas. And why not get someone else in the household to cook? If your kids are old enough, give them a day a week when dinner is their responsibility or make sure your partner cooks whenever they can. Parenting is a marathon, not a sprint, and trying to be good all the time just leads to burnout. It is all about finding a way to be a parent that is sustainable, and this involves having a strong 'good enough' principle rather than aiming for perfection.

Sharing the load

Try to get children involved from an early age. Small children can weigh out pasta, mix a salad, or just take their plates through to the kitchen once they have finished. When they are old enough, get them to stack the dishwasher or do the washing up. And when they are of age, make the rule that 'whoever cooks doesn't do the washing up'. Little bits of help here and there make the whole process more manageable and stop the resentment from brewing up. It also sets good habits for adulthood.

Making it your space

Some mums like to have their children help with chopping or mixing and be involved with mealtimes. But I think it is also nice to have some space and be on my own. So, get the children occupied next door, put your music on, and revel in the peace! If cooking also becomes a moment of space, then it will feel like less of a chore.

In summary

A key part of good food parenting is managing the home environment. This means providing healthy food for your child so that they can eat it. They cannot eat what is not there! Yet, life is busy; we are tired and preparing complicated, delicious meals can be expensive, time-consuming, demanding, and even dull! But it is still best to cook when we can. This section has offered several ways to cut corners, maintain highish but not high standards and stay sane. It is always better to cook good enough food all the time than perfect food once in a blue moon when you have the time to do it. Do have a look at the recipes at the end of the book.

WHAT SHOULD I DO IF MY CHILD DOES NOT LIKE HEALTHY FOOD?

Chapter 1 described how a child's diet should be high in fruit and vegetables, high in complex carbohydrates, such as brown bread, brown pasta and brown rice, and relatively low in fat and sugary foods. It should also be low in salt and very low in ultra-processed foods. This chapter has also described how to cook 'good enough' healthy food even if you have little time. So how can you apply good food parenting to a child who doesn't seem to like healthy food? Children often announce food preferences out of the blue and say, 'I don't like peas', 'I don't like potatoes', and 'I don't like fruit'. Here are some basic strategies for making sure your children eat plenty of fruit and vegetables, a diet high in complex carbohydrates and relatively low in fat. I have also included some tips on how to limit the sugary foods they eat. These tips reflect the ways in which we learn what to eat (Chapter 2) and use the good food parenting strategies of being a good role model, saying the right things and managing their environment.

How do I get them to eat more fruit?

Eating fruit is good for children, even between meals. It helps them grow, concentrate, and develop a healthy mind and body. Here are some simple ways to get them to eat more.

Buy fruit

Buy fruit and bring it into the house! Children like to graze and grab food when they are hungry. If there are bags of crisps around, they will grab those. But if there is fruit, then this is what they will find when they are hungry. Grapes, satsumas, small bananas, and small apples are particularly popular as they are easy to hold and carry around and are about the right size for small hands.

Get a fruit bowl

Buy grapes, satsumas, small bananas, and apples and place them in a fruit bowl. Then put the fruit bowl in a central place where your children can reach it whenever they feel hungry. Ideally, this is somewhere where they walk past regularly and at a child's level. Snacking between meals is not a great habit to get into, but eating fruit between meals is fine and a good way to get children to eat fruit when they are feeling hungry. Just make sure they clean their teeth properly, as I know dentists have a problem with fruit!

Use mindless eating in a good way

Try giving your child a bowl of chopped-up fruit when they are watching TV. Make it a treat; put it in a nice bowl and say, 'Here's a lovely fruit bowl for you', and watch it disappear as they make their way through it without thinking. People often show 'mindless eating' and eat food without really registering it. This can make people overeat as they eat according to the size of the portion or whether it is there rather than whether or not they are actually hungry. That is why we eat all the 'grab bag' of crisps rather than just the smaller 30 g we used to eat. But for children, we can make use of mindless eating and giving them a bowl of fruit whilst they are in the car, busy watching TV or playing a computer game is an easy way to improve their diet.

Make fruit your pudding

Try not to have puddings after every meal, but occasionally, have a special treat of pudding (say twice a week) and make sure this has fruit in it. This could be fruit crumble, fruit and custard, fruit and yoghurt, fruit cake, or just a chopped-up pineapple or mango. But make it seem special so that the fruit is seen as a treat.

Packed lunches

If your child has packed lunches, then make sure, every day, that this has some form of fruit in it. Grapes are the easiest in a little pot, but an apple, satsuma, or banana is also good. Even if they do not eat it every day, persist as they will start to learn that a lunch is not complete unless it consists of fruit as well as everything else.

Drink it

Nowadays, there are a number of ways to drink fruit. Buy fruit juice rather than squash; water it down if it is too strong, and give your children a glass with their breakfast. Dentists suggest drinking juice only with meals to protect teeth, and watered-down juice is less acidic. I personally prefer my children to drink water with their lunch and dinner, as I do not think all meals should be made to be sweet. So, I would recommend juice for breakfast and water for other meals. There are also fruit smoothies, fruit cartons, and fruit sachets, which are an easy way to get children to eat fruit. But do not overdo these, as they are bad for teeth. In addition, drinks that are actually food and contain quite a lot of calories are not a good habit to get into, as the calorie content of a drink is less likely to be registered than if it is eaten as a food. This can encourage overeating as people forget the 'drinks' they have had, which are actually 'meals'. This is OK for small children, but as adults, we live in a world of high-calorie drinks from many different popular fast-food outlets and may not realise that the 'drink' actually counts as food and is adding to our energy intake. It is always better to eat food than drink it.

How do I get them to eat more vegetables?

Children need a variety of vegetables in their diet. Here are some ways to get them to eat more.

Buy vegetables

You are in charge of the money, the shopping, and the cooking. They are not. So buy vegetables and bring them into the house. Then give them to your children. They cannot eat vegetables if they are not on offer. Always have a supply of frozen peas, beans, and broccoli in the freezer and a cucumber and carrots in the fridge. Children seem to like these the most, so always give these at meals. If you are trying a new vegetable, give it as well as one they like, so at least they get something, and this takes the pressure off having to eat something different.

Persist

Make sure every meal has vegetables with it. Even if they get left, persist and keep giving them to your child. Eventually, they will give in, AND they will learn that a meal is not complete unless it consists of some sort of vegetable. If they say, 'I don't like broccoli', still put one piece on their plate. One day, they will just eat it. This is particularly effective if they have a friend round for tea. If their friend eats their broccoli, your child will too.

Be a good role model

Eat with your children as much as possible, and comment on how nice the vegetables are. So do not say, 'Eat your beans, they are good for you'. Say, 'Have some beans, they are really juicy'. Then be seen to eat your own vegetables and enjoy them.

Raw vegetables

Many children prefer their vegetables raw and crunchy. So, give them uncooked carrots or peppers, even if you are eating yours cooked.

Make them a treat

Frozen peas in a bowl in front of the TV will get eaten mindlessly. If you say, 'Would you like a lovely bowl of frozen peas?', they will feel that they are being treated and eat their vegetables without even noticing.

Hide them

Many mums hide vegetables in their food, so children eat them without even knowing they are doing so. Use tomato-based sauces whenever you can; grate carrots into spaghetti bolognese and add finely chopped onions and peppers in shepherd's pie.

Use peer pressure

When they are going to a friend's for tea, never tell the mum, 'they don't like xxx', and when the mum asks, 'What do they like?' always answer, 'Feed them whatever you were going to cook'. Children may well not eat cauliflower, broccoli, or beans at home, but strangely, will wolf them down when at a friend's house. Likewise, when you have children back home for tea, give all the children the same food and even use it as a time to cook a food you know your child says they do not like. If their friend eats it, then they may well eat it as well.

Let them choose

If you take your kids shopping, then let them choose a new vegetable as a treat. Then cook it, and they might be more likely to try it if they have chosen it.

Catch them when they are hungry

Before tea, my children become 'fridge magnets' and start hanging around, looking for food. Take advantage of this and give them a bowl of frozen peas or carrot sticks to munch on.

Drink them

Nowadays, there are vegetable juices that children like. Give them these for their packed lunch. But do not be overly reliant on drinking. As with fruit, it is always better to eat food than drink it, as that way, the food gets registered as food, and we feel fuller afterwards. Drinks can have hidden calories and can prompt overeating if people do not realise that the drink they had in the car was actually half a meal.

How do I get them to eat complex carbohydrates?

Children need a diet high in complex carbohydrates to give them energy and help them grow. Complex carbohydrates most commonly come in the form of bread, potatoes, pasta, and rice, and should form the main ingredient of any meal. As a rule, BROWN is far better than white, as brown bread, brown pasta, or brown rice releases its energy more slowly, filling us up for longer and sustaining us between meals. So, how do you get your child to eat BROWN complex carbohydrates?

Buy them

Children can only eat the food you buy. So, buy brown bread, brown pasta, and brown rice and bring them into your house. If your children are very small, then just feed them these from the start, and they will never know that there is an alternative. Brown should be the norm, and they will like them, eat them, and comment when other people eat the horrible white versions.

Do not mention it

At its simplest, if you do not mention that the pasta, rice, or bread is now brown, then children will not notice the difference. They actually do not taste that different, particularly when covered in sauce or toasted and buttered.

Mix it up

If you feel that your children are more sensitive to such things, then mix it up for a while. Cook pasta that is half white and half brown and see how they get on. You could mix it in with orange, green, and brown pasta, so it is all just a different colour, and the chances are they will eat it. Nowadays, there is even wholemeal bread that looks white that you could use. Then, after a while, tell them: 'By the way, that's brown bread you've been eating', and shift to the proper thing.

Be a good role model

Do not say, 'We are going to eat brown bread as it's healthier'. Health does not really work as a motivation for children, as it is too long-term, and they live in the present. Be positive and say, 'This bread is much more filling' or, 'This pasta goes much better with this sauce' or, 'This rice is much less mushy than the other rice' or just 'Ooh, this is lovely'. Then eat your food with pleasure in front of them.

Make it the norm.

Children eat what is given to them and what they are familiar with. Do not offer them a choice; just always buy and cook brown foods, and they will eat them. Even cook them when other children come for tea, and eat them yourself. And when you eat out, if the pasta or bread is white, do not say, 'Ooh, what a treat! White bread at last', say, 'This is much less tasty than what we have at home'.

Choose the version most similar to what they are used to.

If they have always eaten sliced white bread, it will be more difficult to introduce a dense, seeded home meal loaf, so start with a sliced wholemeal loaf that looks and feels more like what they are used to. Similarly, start with fine brown rice rather than a thick nutty one and brown pasta, which is similar in shape to their normal one. This way, they probably will not even notice the difference. But if they do complain, persist and make positive noises about how nice it is whilst you eat it.

Persistence.

Keeping going is always the key. Children like what they know and know what they get. And some do not like change. But if you just persist, very soon, what they know will shift, and so will what they like, particularly if you eat with them and show them that you like the food you want them to eat.

Potatoes

Officially, according to nutritionists, potatoes are not complex carbohydrates but simple carbohydrates. They therefore release their energy quickly and don't keep us as full as complex carbohydrates. BUT I think the simple potato has a very important role in our diet and is full of vitamins and minerals (and has been since it was brought all the way back from South America!). So, eat potatoes in all their form throughout your week, but try to mix it up and have boiled, mashed, jacket potatoes, as well as chips.

Be varied

Each meal should have a complex carbohydrate in it for energy and growth. But mix it up and make sure you use potatoes, rice, pasta and bread across your meals to stop your children getting bored and to give them the variety they need.

How do I encourage them to eat less fat?

After the age of 5, children should eat a diet relatively low in fat. This does NOT mean a low-fat diet. It means a diet whereby fat makes up a smaller percentage than carbohydrates, fruit or vegetables. So how can this be achieved?

Naturally low-fat foods

Many foods are naturally low in fat. In fact, pretty much all fruits and all vegetables, brown bread, brown pasta and brown rice, potatoes, fish, pulses (chickpeas and lentils) and water (!) have no or a very low amount of fat in them. Therefore, eating a low-fat diet simply means eating lots of fruits and vegetables and complex carbohydrates. If you do this, then your diet will be low in fat.

Adding fat

But we do not just eat bread, pasta, rice, and potatoes; we add fat, and have toast and butter, pasta and cheese, rice and curry, and chips cooked in oil. This is completely fine as long as your child's diet is still mostly fruit, vegetables, and complex carbohydrates. Therefore, have toast with some butter (not loads), have pasta (with some cheese), mostly rice (with some curry) and eat your potatoes boiled, mashed in their jackets, as well as having chips sometimes.

Protein, meat, and fish

Children need protein in their diets, and a good source is meat and fish. Most meat can easily be made to be low(ish) in fat by simply cutting the fat off. Then try to cook it without adding much fat back in. Grilled, baked, or shallow-fried with a small amount of oil is better than deep-fried with lots of oil. Fish is mostly naturally low in fat and stays that way if it is not always wrapped in butter and fried. Reduce the frequency of processed meats such as bacon, sausages, and ham, as they contain high levels of salt and other preservatives, which may be harmful. Also, only eat smoked foods occasionally, as they also may be damaging in large quantities.

Low-fat alternatives

The food industry now produces 'low-fat' versions of practically every food, including fat. But be suspicious. To make milk low in fat, they simply take the fat out. But to make prepared ready meals 'low fat', the fat may well come out, but other things are added in, including sugar, artificial fats, or salt. So, I personally buy low-fat milk but avoid other more unnatural 'low-fat' foods. If you make your own shepherd's pie, pasta, and tomato sauce or chicken stew, then it will be low in fat if you do not add much fat back in. If you buy the processed 'low-fat' versions, they may be low in fat, but chances are they are very high in something else.

How do I reduce sugary foods?

Children do not need sweets, cakes, biscuits, or chocolate to grow and develop. They are not a necessary part of the diet, and if they had never been invented, children would be fine. They can cause an instant reduction in hunger, which is useful if your child feels starving, but very quickly that sugar high will drop dramatically, and your child will feel hungrier than they did before and want more. BUT they exist, and children (mostly) like them, and parents like to give them. So how should they be managed?

Keep them out of the house

You shop and cook, and choose what comes into the house. If you keep sugary foods out of the house, then children cannot pester you for them, and you cannot be tempted to use them to make your child behave.

Choose sugary foods that are foods

Cakes and biscuits are proper foods with sugar in them. They have a place in our diets and add to our nutritional intake. Sweets and chocolates are not 'food'. They are just sugar. Give your child food that is sweet rather than just sweets. And try to give them sugary foods that also contain fruit or complex carbohydrates, such as oat-based bars or biscuits, fruit crumble, fruit puddings, or fruit yoghurts.

Don't make them too special

If you give your child a biscuit and say, 'Aren't you lucky?' or, 'You have been a good little boy', then they will see biscuits as special, exciting and a treat. If you share a large ice cream pudding and bond over how wonderful it is, they will see ice cream as a time to be close to their mum and a way to feel good about themselves. But if puddings are mostly fruit-based, and when they are not, they are just another course at the end of a meal, they can be enjoyed, but without being given the extra special status as being more important and nicer than the savoury foods they have just eaten.

Don't make them forbidden

BUT do not ban sugary foods from your child; otherwise, they will simply see them as even more special and even more exciting. Sweets exist in the world, and your child will eat them. If you ban them, when they grow up and want to rebel, then food will start to become the perfect way to react against you and make you cross.

Fit them into your life

Have food-based sugary foods such as cakes and biscuits at home, occasionally. But have sweets and chocolate outside of the home, as part of your routine on an occasional basis. A weekly trip to the sweet shop on the way home from school stops sweets from becoming forbidden or too special, but keeps them limited and attached to a specific time and place. Or a chocolate cake after lunch at the weekend in your favourite café, let them have what they want, stop them pestering you for it for the rest of the week, and give it a place in their diet, which is limited.

In summary

Children need a varied diet, high in fruit and vegetables and brown complex carbohydrates, with a moderate amount of meat and fish and a small amount of fat and sugar. The best way to achieve this is to cook as much as you can and buy and cook the food you want your children to eat. Persist with healthy food, and if at first your child declares they do not like it, try to make it the norm. And be a good role model by eating healthy food in front of them and saying how nice it is. Also, try tricks such as giving them fruit and vegetables to eat when they are busy doing something else, cook puddings that are fruit and contain real food, hide vegetables in their food if you have to and allow them to have some sweets outside of the home so as not to make them forbidden.

In conclusion

We have to eat, and we have to feed our children. This can feel like a real chore, and often, people feel that they just do not have time to cook. Hopefully, this chapter has illustrated how cooking for a family does not need to take up too much time or effort and that if you shop for ingredients rather than meals, it is possible to rustle up a meal that is healthy and filling (even if not very exciting), and still keep your sanity. It has also illustrated how you can use good food parenting by being a good role model, saying the right things and managing a child's environment to encourage your child to eat a healthy diet and develop a positive relationship with food.

REFERENCE

1. Ogden, J. (2014). The good parenting food guide: Managing what children eat without making food a problem. Oxford: Wiley Blackwell. Made Open Access (2021). https://openresearch.surrey.ac.uk/esploro/outputs/book/The-Good-Parenting-Food-Guide/99604423802346

4

WHAT SHOULD I DO IF MY CHILD EATS TOO MUCH OR TOO LITTLE?

If food were just a matter of biology, we would eat when we were hungry and stop when we were full. Unfortunately, our worlds sometimes seem to conspire to make us eat too much and become overweight or eat too little and become fussy or develop disordered eating. This is worrying for parents who want to encourage their children to eat less (if they overeat) or more (if they undereat), but without doing harm. This chapter will explore how to manage a child who either eats too much or too little without making food into a problem. It is never about putting a child on a diet or pressurising them to eat, but about drawing up the pillars of being a good role model, saying the right things and managing their environment.

WHAT SHOULD I DO IF MY CHILD EATS TOO MUCH?

We live in a modern world where portion sizes are getting bigger and obesity is on the increase. If you feel that your child eats too much and is becoming overweight, then it might be time to do something. This chapter will describe how you can decide whether

DOI: 10.4324/9781003600183-8

or not you should be worrying about your child. Then, if you should be, it next describes some tips to encourage them to eat less. BUT do not put them on a diet, as this might make them think about food even more and store up more serious weight problems for later on in life. The last thing you want is to make food into an issue.

Decide if you need to worry

I do not agree with having bathroom scales in a house with children, as it can make them overly worried about their weight, and weight can become the goal rather than health. But, at times, it can be good to have some hard data and to know if your child is of normal weight or not. Weigh your child when you can, but do it casually without making it a big deal. If you are staying at someone else's house who has scales, in the local chemist's or at the train station, get everyone to jump on the scales 'for fun' and see what they weigh. Next, a few days later, in response to someone saying something about height, 'Mum, have I grown?', 'Tom's taller than me now' or even, 'My shoes don't fit', stand them against the wall and measure their height. Then use the charts available online to find out their Body Mass Index (BMI) without saying anything to them. If their weight is normal, they are fine, and you can ignore how much they eat. If they are underweight, read the next section. But if they are overweight, they may be developing a weight problem.

Also consider the following questions:

- Is your child anxious around food?
- Are they overly concerned with how they look?
- Do they ever sneak food from the cupboards when you are not around?
- Do they refuse to eat at mealtimes, then eat on their own later in a guilty way (i.e. at night, in the garden, in their bedroom)?

If your child is overweight and you have answered yes to any of the above, then your child might be developing an eating problem. If this is the case, then take them to the doctor, as all the evidence indicates that early diagnosis and treatment are the best way forward. If they are just a bit overweight, then here are some tips for helping them to eat less without making food an issue.

Do not put them on a diet

Being a bit overweight as a child is not great. But developing a problem with eating as a child may lead to a lifetime of worry and depression. If you think your child is over-eating, then try all the tips below to get their eating back on track, but do not put them on a diet. Going on a diet ultimately means having to deny yourself foods that you want to eat. This can make those foods seem even more tempting and, in the end, when people break their diet (which most do), they eat even more than they would have done before. So, limit your child's food in subtle ways by being a good role model, changing what food you buy and cook and planning meals so that they can learn to live with their hunger. But if you put them on a diet, you may well make the situation worse, and food will become even more of a treat than it ever was. And as time goes on, you may have set your child up for a future of struggling with one of the central parts of day-to-day life.

Be more active

Becoming overweight is a balance between energy in (food) and energy out (activity). If you think your child is becoming overweight, the simplest way forward is to get them to be more active. Chapter 5 covers this in depth, but go for walks or family bike rides at weekends; rather than watching a film, buy them a ball and a skipping rope, throw them out in the garden or street to play, take them to the local park, encourage them to join clubs at school and show them that you like being active as well. And say the right things about exercise, such as, 'Go out in the garden and let off some steam', 'I'm tired, I think I'll go for a walk' and 'That bike ride has made me feel so much better'.

Be a good role model for eating

You are your child's key role model for most of their childhood, so be a good role model for eating. Eat healthily, eat meals and do not snack; do not skip meals and have seconds if you are hungry, but not if you just feel like it.

Be a good role model for body size

Also, be a good role model for body size. We live in a world where people are getting fatter, and being overweight has become the norm. If you are overweight, do not let your child think that this is how they should be. And DO NOT encourage them to think that being overweight runs in your family and that there is nothing you can do about it. Do not moan to your child about your weight, but also do not celebrate it. Similarly, if they are overweight, do not criticise them for it, but also do not make it something to be proud of.

Say the right things

Being a good role model involves saying the right things to give your child some healthy scripts in their head for the future. So do not say, 'We are all fat in our family. It's just the way we are', as they will believe being overweight is beyond their control and inevitable. Also, do not say, 'I'm so fat. I hate it. It's so ugly', or even, 'You are getting fat. You'll have no friends'. Such criticisms lead to low self-esteem, self-criticism, and possibly comfort eating, which all make the problem even worse. And do not comment on their eating, saying: 'You eat so much', 'Gosh, you can put it away', 'You have such a huge appetite' or 'You never seem to be full', as these phrases will stick with them and they will start to see them as true and a core part of who they are. Similarly, do not praise them saying, 'My lovely fat daughter', 'You are so fat and cuddly' or 'It's so nice having someone chubby to cuddle up to', as they will believe they need to stay overweight in order to be loved. Mostly, it is best to say nothing! But if you are talking about eating and body size, do it about someone else in a more neutral way. So, when you see a celebrity of a healthy size, say: 'She looks lovely', and when a friend comes round who is of a healthier weight, say: 'She looks really healthy'; positively praise being active and eating well by saying: 'Let's go for a bike ride this weekend. That will be fun', and 'This casserole is really nice'.

Change their environment

Until the age of about 12, you are completely in charge of what your child eats as you shop, drive the car, have the money and do the cooking. Even after this age, most of what they eat is still up to you. So, the best way to encourage them to eat less is to change their environment by only buying healthy foods and bringing them into the house. Do not buy fizzy drinks, crisps or biscuits if you do not want your children to eat them and cook healthy meals without puddings. And give them decent portions, but do not overload them with their first serving, so that they have to ask if they want more rather than just eating everything that is in front of them. Then, without them realising it, they will snack less and eat well, and food will not become an issue.

Portion control

Strangely enough, a large plate half empty feels less than a small plate full of food! So, if you feel your child is overeating and you want to limit how much they eat, make sure that you have reasonably sized plates. And all have the same plates! That way, you all will be able to eat a decent-sized meal and be able to empty your plate without feeling deprived.

Plan meals

Children get hungry and will graze on whatever is available. But if there is a set time for meals when they know that they will reliably be fed, living with the hunger and waiting for the next meal becomes easier. So, decide to eat at a set time whenever possible, tell your children when and what you are having for tea and ask them to wait, saying, 'It is much nicer to be hungry at teatime. You'll enjoy it more'.

Cook filling meals

If your child is hungry, they will eat in between meals. They will then eat less at mealtimes, be hungry shortly afterwards and eat in between meals. It is a vicious cycle. So, cook meals that are substantial and filling. Make sure there is plenty of carbohydrate (brown pasta, rice or bread) to fill them up and plenty of vegetables and protein. Do not cook foods that are high in fat, as these may fill them up in the short term, but this will not last. And avoid sugary foods, as this will give them an immediate sugar high and a sense of fullness, which will quickly drop right down, making them want more sugar to get the high back again.

Eat breakfast

Breakfast is such an important meal as it kick-starts the metabolism, gets us out of the hibernation state we have been in overnight and sets us up for the day. If we miss it, we stay sluggish and cannot concentrate until lunchtime. So set out breakfast every morning, sit down with the children and make breakfast a normal part of the daily routine. And also get them to drink something!

Eat as a family

Eating as a family is the easiest way to set up what is healthy and that healthy is normal. So, eat as a family as often as you can and then you can be a good role model, say the right things, serve out the right food in the right-sized portions and help to make eating a normal and stress-free part of the family day.

Seize a moment to have a chat

At some point, it would be good to have a chat about being overweight and the dangers associated with overeating. But as with talking about undereating (see the next section), if you lecture your child over dinner or nag them in the car, they will switch off, ignore you and get cross. So be more subtle and underhanded, and seize the moment in a more casual way. When you see someone on the TV who is overweight, say: 'That can't be healthy, being that size', or when a celebrity is shown having gained a huge amount of weight, say: 'Did you know that being overweight can shorten your life'. But do not focus on the hugely obese featured in all the programmes designed to shock, as no one relates to these images, and they can make people feel like: 'Well, I'm OK as I'm not as big as them'.

Get a fruit bowl

Sometimes, children get so hungry they cannot last between meals, and the best snack available is fruit. Buy a fruit bowl and fill it with fruit, and place it in a central place so they can help themselves whenever they walk by. This way, they will not need unhealthy snacks but will still be hungry enough when the meal is ready.

In summary

If you think your child eats too much and is overweight, first find out whether you really need to worry. If they are overweight and seem to be developing a problem with food, then seek help, as this is beyond the scope of this book. However, if they just seem to eat too much then do not put them on a diet but try to make them more active, do become a good role model, say the right things about food, change their environment without them realising it, plan meals so that they know when food is coming and seize the moment in a casual way to have a chat about the problems with being overweight. But do all this in an indirect, non-confrontational way, as the last thing you want to do is make food into an issue and set them off into a future of eating problems.

WHAT SHOULD I DO IF MY CHILD EATS TOO LITTLE?

Most children in the Western world are far more likely to end up overweight than underweight, and the most common worry is that a child is eating too much. Some parents, however, do worry that their child is underweight and undereating. This section will first describe how you can decide whether to worry about how much your child is eating. It will next describe some tips for how to manage a child who you feel is not eating enough, BUT without making food into an issue for them.

Work out what is normal

The first step is to work out what a normal weight and a normal healthy food intake are, and to decide whether you need to worry. Babies' weights are often checked against height/weight charts that come from bottle-fed babies in the 1960s, and can make health visitors and parents panic that their baby is not thriving. Food portions are getting bigger, and children are getting fatter, causing a shift in what is considered normal, so a skinny (but healthy) child of the 1960s may well look like they are malnourished and underweight today. Teenagers can suddenly shoot up and stretch, making them look like bean poles that need feeding up. And fatter children, or parents of fatter children, may well comment that your child is skinny and in need of a good meal. But all of this does not mean that your child is underweight. It is just a sign of a changing world and the ways in which our notion of a healthy body size has shifted over the past few decades. In order to make a proper judgement, ask yourself the following questions:

- Is my child's BMI in the normal weight range? (Measure your child's height and weight, but do not make a big thing of it. Wait until you are at someone's house with some scales and get everyone to jump on for the fun of it. Then, a few days later, suggest you measure everyone's height).
- Do they seem unwell and more tired than usual?
- Do they seem anxious around food?
- Are they finding excuses not to eat?
- Are they becoming overly concerned with how they look?
- Are they refusing some foods but still eating lots of their favourite foods if you cook them?

You should worry if your child's BMI is below the normal weight range, if they seem unwell, anxious around food, if they avoid eating with you and if they are overly worried about how they look. Then you should take them to your doctor. But if they are just a bit skinny and going through a fussy stage, when they will eat plenty if you cook what they like, but announce that they don't like the rest, then the best way forward is to ignore it and see it as a stage they will grow out of. In general, here are some tips for getting your child to eat more without making food into an issue.

Be a good role model for eating

Children of all ages learn what and how much to eat from their parents. Up until the age of about 12, parents are their key role models. After this age, even if it starts to feel that their friends are more important and that we are losing our grip, secretly, they still watch what their parents do, and, whether they like it or not, they will probably end up like us. So the most important thing you can do is to be a good role model. Eat healthy foods, do not snack, do not overeat or undereat and be seen to try new foods and enjoy them.

Be a good role model for body satisfaction

Be a good role model for how you feel about how you look. If you have issues with your own body size, then being a parent is about putting these to one side and not letting your child know about them. Don't complain about being too fat or too thin to your child, don't discuss going on the latest diet, don't comment on the body weight of their friends or your friends and don't point to a celebrity in a magazine and say 'I would love to look like that!' Celebrate other aspects of yourself and your child, making the most of how clever, funny, kind, hard-working, sporty or creative they are. And make them realise that how they look is only one aspect of who they are.

Eat as a family

Try to eat at the table with the family as often as you can. Eating with others can make eating seem more normal and less of an issue, as the focus is less on the food and more on the conversation. But do not make the mealtime a chance to nag your child about homework, delve into their private lives or argue with your partner. Make mealtimes as easy as possible and a fairly neutral time when people can get together to eat and chat.

Say the right things

What you say is almost as important as what you do. So say the right things about food and body size. Eat healthy food and comment 'this is lovely', have a second helping, saying: 'This is really lovely', and stop when you are full, saying: 'I am full now'. Do not call healthy food 'boring' or even 'so healthy'. Do not say: 'I'm still hungry but I must not eat anymore, in case I get fat' and do not comment: 'I'm stuffed but I'll just have one more portion'. Try to talk about food in a way that reinforces eating when you are hungry and stopping when you are full, and does not make body size an issue.

Do not focus on the food

If your child is undereating and going through a stage of refusing food, do not make their eating behaviour the focus of the family. First, do not ask them: 'Would you like some potatoes' or 'We are having spaghetti bolognese. Is that OK?' This can make them feel too much in control and give them too much choice. Cook food you know they like without asking them. Next, place it on their plate the same as everyone else in the family. Then all chat, including them in the conversation, but without making them the focus of the meal. You may find that by the end of the meal, they have eaten what they were given without even thinking about it. Sometimes, ignoring a problem does make it go away, whereas focusing on it gives it the attention that the child was after.

Be encouraging

You can encourage a child to eat more, but do not let this dominate a meal. The odd comment, such as 'try and eat a few more peas' or 'have a bit more of your tea or you'll be hungry later on', is fine. But pressure, blackmail, anger, upset and any kind of drama will make your child dig in their heels, and you will have lost the battle. The key saying to parenting is 'pick your fights carefully'. If you say, 'You are not leaving the table until you have finished your tea', then you may well have a child still sitting there on their own in the middle of the night. And that is not good for anyone!

Cook what they like

Ideally, children should eat what everyone else eats and be flexible enough to fit in with the family. Also, ideally, parents should offer their children a varied diet, so they get to try new foods and get a proper balance of nutrients. But if your child is going through a fussy stage and starts to declare that they do not like what you cook, then take the pressure off for a while and cook what you know they like. If they like fish fingers, pizza or even the dreaded chicken nuggets (!), cook them (for all the family!) for a few days to take the pressure off and remove the focus from food. Ideally, still try to all eat the same, otherwise they may like the attention of being different and do it casually without a fuss, explaining: 'We are running out of food', or 'I feel like a quick tea tonight'. It is not great to feed your child unhealthy food. But it is far worse to make food an issue. So burst the bubble by giving them what they like, and after a week or so, see if the tension has lifted and go back to your normal way of eating.

Keep it varied

When children go through a fussy stage, it is easy to give them what they like, then get stuck and feed them the same foods again. But try to remember that children do announce random likes and dislikes, which will disappear as quickly as they arrived. Try not to get stuck in a rut and quickly get back into the habit of offering a varied diet again.

Use mindless eating

Mindless eating is usually seen as a problem, and many people mindlessly eat more because it is there. But it can also be used to help children eat healthier foods. So, when your child is watching the TV, give them a bowl of chopped up fruit or a plate of bread, carrot sticks and cucumber, and they will eat it without thinking.

Seize the moment to have a chat

If your child is not eating enough, at some point, it is good to have a chat about eating disorders and how serious they are. You need to emphasise that anorexia has a very high mortality rate and that bingeing can cause long-term harm. But if you lecture them at the dinner table or in the car, they will switch off, ignore you and get cross. The trick is to be more subtle and manipulative! Wait for a time when the subject can come up in a more natural way. This might be due to something on the TV, in a magazine or something they are covering at school. That way, when a character in a sitcom develops an eating disorder, you can say, 'Anorexia is scary. Did you know it can cause infertility and is more likely to kill you than any other mental health problem?' If you are browsing through social media together, say: 'Look at her; she is so thin. She looks dreadful. She'll kill herself if she's not careful'. Or even play 'The Carpenters' and mention that Karen Carpenter died from anorexia and how tragic this was. This may open up a conversation about your child's eating. But if it does not, that is fine, as the seed has been planted, and you can revisit it another time.

Question what is happening at school

Sometimes, problems with friends, schoolwork, teachers or bullying can cause children to eat less at home. Ask your child how things are going and watch for signs with their friends, or ask the teachers to see if there are any problems. Most schools now have excellent pastoral support systems in place, which I have always found really helpful. So go into school and speak to someone. And make sure your child has plenty of opportunities to talk to you. Sometimes, this can be easiest when you are out walking, doing the washing up or at bedtime when things are calmer and less intense than over dinner. 'Sideways talking' can be a lot more useful with children than face-to-face talking!

Question what is happening in the family

The family is a system, and when one family member starts to have problems, it is often because of something someone else has done. For example, if parents are arguing a lot, then a child might stop eating to put the focus on themselves and help the parents bond together. Or, if one child excels at sport, the other might start refusing to eat to claim back some of the attention. And often, children take on the role of 'good child' or 'bad child' in a family to balance each other out. If your child starts to have problems around food, question what has changed in the family, and then see if you can change it back.

Consider how you can change

It is far easier to change yourself than it is to change someone else. If your child has problems, see if changing what you do ultimately helps to change what they do. If you are focusing on what they eat, then focus on some other aspect of them – their schoolwork, friends and hobbies. If you have tried ignoring their eating behaviour, try encouraging them to eat more with praise, sticker charts or outright bribery. If you cook what you like, then try cooking what they like, and if you always eat as a family, let them have tea in front of the TV for a few days. If you are always in with them, go out more, or if you go out a lot, start staying in. Break the rules and shake things up a bit, and see whether this makes a difference.

Use peer pressure

Children like to be like their friends, so use peer pressure to get their eating back on track. Invite friends round for tea and give them all the same food and the same amount to eat. Or get them to make tea with pizza bases and toppings to choose from, or even let them make whatever they like. Try asking for your child to go to a friend for tea, and tell the mum to feed your child whatever they are feeding theirs, but not to make a fuss about it.

Use natural breaks in the routine

People seem most able to change their behaviour following a life event or life crisis, such as a relationship breakdown, a change of job or a health problem. Although we cannot create life events for our children, times when the normal routine of our lives is challenged, such as family get-togethers, after an illness, holidays or birthdays, can all be a useful time to break any unhealthy habits your child has developed, whether it is under- or overeating. So take advantage of any such events and use them as a chance to get your child to think less about food, worry less about how they look or find a new, healthier approach to eating. But not by making a fuss about what they eat, just by letting the ongoing events shake things up a bit and seeing what happens.

Seek help

Eating disorders are very rare in children under the age of 12, but more common in teenagers, particularly teenage girls. Most of the evidence indicates that early diagnosis and early intervention are best. If your child is losing weight, has a BMI below the normal weight and is starting to become anxious around food, then seek help. I would avoid making food into an issue if your child is just going through a stage or becoming a bit picky about their food. But if your child is developing a problem, professional help way beyond the scope of this book is the best way forward.

In summary

In terms of probabilities, it is more likely that your child will end up overeating and overweight than undereating and underweight. The first stage is to decide whether you really have something to worry about or whether your skinny child just looks skinny due to changing social norms in a world that is getting fatter. But if you are worried and think your child needs to eat more, then this chapter has offered some possible ways to encourage your child to eat more without making food into an issue. These include being a good role model by eating well and not publicly worrying about your own body size, saying the right things about eating and weight, having family meals that are more about chats than food, not making food into the focus of the family, encouraging your child to eat more in a casual non-confrontational way, using mindless eating in positive ways, finding out what is happening at school or in the family, changing your own behaviour, using peer pressure and taking advantage of natural changes in the family routine to make a change. So, **do** find ways to encourage your child to eat more if you feel they genuinely are undereating. But do not make food into an issue, as this could store up even bigger problems for the future.

To conclude

Giving a child the best start involves trying to be a good food parent and helping them to develop a healthy relationship with food. Sometimes, they might eat too much, which can lead to becoming overweight. Sometimes, they can eat too little, leading to weight loss. This chapter has used the three key pillars of good food parenting to address these issues in terms of being a good role model, managing their environment and saying the right things. Together, these approaches can encourage a child to eat well in ways that are both positive and subtle, and avoid many of the more direct approaches that can lead to rebound effects, with children deciding to do the opposite of what you say. This way, you can set them up for life with a good relationship with food, which should help them avoid many of the pitfalls that can challenge them as they go through adulthood.

5

WHAT SHOULD I DO IF MY CHILD HAS POOR BODY IMAGE OR SPENDS TOO MUCH TIME ON THEIR PHONE?

Whilst many parents worry about their child eating too much or too little, there are many other areas that can cause concern. This chapter will explore how to manage a child who has poor body image, focusing on how you can change what you do and say, acknowledge their feelings and move the emphasis away from how they look. It also suggests some practical changes to your home, such as removing the scales and the full-length mirrors. Next, it will offer some tips for encouraging a child to become more active by focusing on the more immediate benefits of exercise, such as having fun and being with friends.

HOW CAN I HELP MY CHILD FEEL BETTER ABOUT HOW THEY LOOK?

Many adults do not like the way they look, and women, in particular, often feel that they are too fat and unattractive. Men can also be dissatisfied with their bodies; they often say that they want to be taller or more muscular. Unfortunately, children nowadays also have

DOI: 10.4324/9781003600183-9

these feelings, and both girls and boys as young as nine have been shown to worry about being fat. But it is not only being too fat that can make them unhappy. Feeling too short, too tall, too skinny, too spotty, having curly hair, having straight hair, or just feeling different in a million possible ways from the way they would like to look can be upsetting. This chapter will offer some tips on how to manage a child who is critical of how they look and suggest some ways to shift their attention away from their bodies onto other aspects of who they are.

Be a good role model

If you criticise how you look to your children, then they will do the same. You are their greatest role model, and if you have issues about your own body image, then being a parent is about trying to put these on one side and presenting a positive front to your child. This is particularly important when they are entering puberty, as any concerns they have will start to burst to the surface as their body changes and grows in ways that can feel scary and confusing. At best, make positive comments about yourself. But if you cannot manage this, then just say nothing!

Say the right things about your child

It is fine to call your child 'pretty', 'beautiful', 'handsome' or 'good looking' sometimes. But try not to make compliments based upon looks, the staple diet of how you speak about them. If your daughter is always 'mummy's pretty girl' or your son 'daddy's handsome boy', then they will grow up valuing how they look above all other aspects of themselves. And then, when they feel that they are no longer 'pretty' or 'handsome', not only will they have that to worry about, but they may also worry that their mum or dad will no longer find them special. So, also comment on what they do and what they are, as well as how they look. Tell them that they are clever, funny, kind, caring, hardworking, good at making friends, and thoughtful and then they will have a whole spectrum of characteristics to build their confidence upon. I sometimes worry that I did not get this balance right! (1).

Say the right things about others

When watching films or TV, reading a book, or just talking about family and friends, try to keep comments about how they look to a minimum. If all comments about celebrities are that they are 'too fat', 'too thin', 'looking old' or 'not as pretty in real life', then your child will learn that looks are key to who we are. But if they hear that this celebrity does a lot of work for charity, or that one is a good actor, then the world can become a more well-rounded place where how we look is just one of many aspects of who we are. At times, this can feel like fighting an impossible battle as we are surrounded by so many fake images of 'beautiful' people. But if your child gets healthy messages at home, then maybe this can undo some of the damage done by all the other sources of information.

Acknowledge their feelings

It is true that some children are fatter than others; that some are shorter than their friends; that many get spots; and that quite a few go through a strange stage in puberty when their jaws grow at different rates to their heads or their legs stretch like strings. If your child does not like the way they look, and you can sort of see the point, then you need to acknowledge their feelings, but then try to get them to reframe them in a more positive way. So, if your child IS fat and says, 'I'm fat', or your child is spotty and says, 'I'm spotty', it is no good saying, 'No, you are not darling; you are lovely'. This may feel as if you are being reassuring, but what you are actually doing is denying their experiences and brushing away their feelings. So, acknowledge their feelings and say, 'Yes, you have put a bit of weight on at the moment' or 'Yes, you are a bit spotty at the moment'. Then say, 'And I guess that must feel a bit difficult'; that way, you are acknowledging what they are going through. Then ask them a bit about it, such as, 'Why do you think that is?' and listen. After a while, try to reframe what they are feeling by doing the following: emphasise that it is a stage they are going through and will probably pass as they grow up; ask for examples of their friends that are also fat/spotty/short, etc. to make them feel that they are not alone; then ask if they know of anyone who went through this stage and came out the other side to make them realise that things change. Hopefully, this will make them feel listened to and that the problem is not as great as they thought. This is similar to the principles of Cognitive Behaviour Therapy (CBT), which can easily be used at home.

Focus on the positives

If they are upset about something about their appearance and you have had a conversation trying to acknowledge their feelings, then a day or so later, start trying to focus on positive aspects of who they are. Be particularly positive about any work they bring home from school or the way they manage their friends. Mention the fact that they made their bed, were kind to their pets or even kind to you. And just try to boost them up in general. Even mention something about their appearance, saying, 'Your hair looks lovely today' or 'Your eyes are so blue'.

Bin the scales

Personally, I have a thing about bathroom scales and think that they are dangerous, particularly for teenagers. So, if you have a child who is starting to worry about how they look (or any child, or, in fact, no child at all!), get rid of the scales. We do not need to know what number the dial says to know whether we have gained or lost weight – our clothes tell us that, or we can go to the GP and be weighed. But that dial in the bathroom can make people obsessed with their weight and have them watching the minute changes, which could easily be due to time of the month, the size of their dinner or how much they have drunk rather than any actual weight loss. If you desperately still need to know how much you weigh, then pop around to a friend's house or to the chemist, but for the sake of your child, I think the scales should go.

Move the mirrors

I also worry about full-length mirrors in children's bedrooms. I have no evidence for this, and I know of no studies that have looked at the effect of mirrors, but I feel that children alone in their rooms, having all the emotions that they have, with a full-length mirror to stare at and scrutinise every aspect of themselves, cannot be healthy. So, have them in communal spaces, but particularly if your child is starting to worry about how they look, move the mirrors and make it that bit harder for them to criticise their bodies. BUT do not do this in a dramatic way, saying, 'I've had enough of you staring at yourself. This has got to go!' Find an excuse, such as: 'We are having a clear out', 'The walls need painting' or 'It's better in the guest room where everyone can use it', then move it without them quite knowing why.

Do not comment on what they wear

There are many fights to have with our children, and the key to parenting is to pick your fights carefully. What they wear or the style or colour of their hair seems to be a fight not worth having. Fashion changes so quickly, and children want to be like their peers, that it is hard for anyone from a different generation to judge what they look like or what signals they are giving out to their peers. If your child looks to you like 'a beggar', 'a thug' or 'a tart', or if your son looks like 'a girl' and your daughter like 'a boy', this may be your interpretation, but what do we know? We are not their peer group. When it comes to fashion, we are well past the age when we can read what it all means anymore. So, it is probably best to keep quiet and save the fight for something more important. And by not commenting on their clothes or their hair, we can teach them the message that how we look is only a small part of what we are about.

Explain the tricks of the media

Every day, we are bombarded with fake images of how people look. Ageing actresses are made to look young, and young, thin, wrinkle-free actresses are made to look even younger, thinner, with pore-less, spotless, perfect skin. This is done through airbrushing, makeup, lighting, body doubles and CGI. Children need to be taught this so that they do not make comparisons between themselves and some-thing that is just not real. It is bad enough comparing yourself to your thinner friend, but at least you know that during PE, their legs wobble and they get spots. But the images in the media present this flawless world, which sets unrealistic goals and makes everyone feel inadequate. So next time you are sitting in a café, find a magazine or have a look at your phone and go through it, showing your children how the images have been changed and emphasising how dangerous this can be.

Use their peer group

The best comparisons to make are always with our peer group. When I worry that I am getting old, I know I will feel old if I look at my stu-dents, but if I compare myself to my same-aged friends, I know I am doing fine. So, when your child is feeling 'short', ask them to tell you the names of two children taller than them. Then, if you know them, list the names of four children, of the same age, who are their height or smaller. Similarly, if they feel spotty, ask them about their friends and see who else has spots. And if they feel fat, make sure you give them a mix of people to focus on who are both thinner and fatter. That way, you can help to take the negativity out of the problem without denying that it exists.

Challenge their beliefs

When children are feeling rotten about themselves, they are prone to make grand generalisations, saying, 'Everyone says I'm fat', 'no one likes me', 'I have no friends' and 'Everyone is thinner than me'. When they do this, help them to change their beliefs by challenging what they think and finding evidence to contradict it. Say, 'Who says you are fat?' Then, after they have listed a few names, say, 'What about Amy? (as you know, she wouldn't). Does she call you fat? What about Emily or Becca?' And say, 'So, who do you sit with at lunch? Do they like you?' or 'You were invited to Tom's party. He must like you'. That way, it is hard for them to hang on to their black and white view of the world, and they have to start to see that it is not as bad as they thought it was. This is also similar to the principles of Cognitive Behaviour Therapy.

Give them a 'good enough' principle

Children and adults who are prone to perfectionism can turn this inwards and start becoming critical of the way they look. As a result, they no longer just want to be the best at school or the best at sports and find it difficult when they make mistakes, they also want to look 'perfect'. If your child is a perfectionist, challenge this as early as you can by celebrating when they 'only' get 16 out of 20 in a test, when they come third in a race or when they are picked as a reserve for the team. In addition, do not worry if they wear odd socks, if their clothes do not seem to match or if their hair gets untidy. And treat yourself in the same way, so that they see you without make-up, see others seeing you this way and hear you being happy with the way you look. Perfectionism can be crippling to both children and adults, and giving them a 'good enough' principle is about the best gift you have to offer.

Seize the moment to have a word about eating problems

If your child is becoming overly worried about their body size, then you need to have a chat about eating disorders and how dangerous they are. But do not do this in a confrontational way, as you rip their mirror out of their bedroom or over dinner. Do it in a subtle 'sideways' way when you are out walking, in a cafe or when prompted by something on the TV or in a magazine. So, do not say, 'You must stop worrying about your size. It could be dangerous'. But do say, 'Gosh, look at her. She's so thin. That's really dangerous. People die from eating disorders, you know'.

Be more active

Teenage girls, in particular, can become extremely inactive and easily spend their days lying around in their rooms doing their hair or texting their friends. If they are worried about how they look, this can make them worry more and become even more focused on their appearance. One of the best solutions is simply to get out more and be more active. Try doing more things as a family that involve getting out of the house and going places, whether it be swimming, bowling, going for a walk or just wandering around the shops. That way, they will be less able to think about themselves and will get distracted, at least for a while (see the next section).

Expand their interests

Try also to get them to take up new hobbies on their own. New clubs or skills will help to build their confidence and shift their attention away from themselves, but choose wisely, as some sports, such as ballet or gymnastics, are very body and mirror focused. Also, get them to do something useful involving helping others. If they are old enough, get them to volunteer at the local soup kitchen, a home for the elderly, with guides, brownies or scouts or at a charity shop. Helping others is a great way to take anyone's attention away from not liking themselves.

In summary

Growing up can be a difficult time, particularly during puberty and adolescence, when a child's body changes in ways that can be upsetting and scary. If your child starts to criticise the way they look, whether it be feeling fat, spotty, too short or too tall, this chapter has offered some tips for moving the attention onto other aspects of who they are. In particular, being a good role model and saying the right things about body size can help them to see that we are more than just how we look. Binning the scales and moving full-length mirrors are simple, practical ways that might help, and encouraging them to be more active and take up new activities and hobbies can expand their horizons. And teach them about the tricks of the media and the ways in which the images we see are fake and unreal. But you also need to acknowledge their feelings and make them feel heard, so do not just offer bland reassurances, but listen to them and then try to focus on the positive aspects of who they are.

HOW CAN I GET MY CHILD TO BE MORE ACTIVE?

Exercise is clearly linked with body weight, and being inactive is central to the development and maintenance of obesity as well as other health problems, such as diabetes, arthritis, bone density, immune function, joint problems and heart disease. Exercise also has many psychological benefits and can help with anxiety, depression, self-esteem, body image, stress management, confidence and friendship problems. Current recommendations suggest that adults should do at least 30 minutes of at least moderate physical activity on at least five days a week, and that children should exercise for at least 60 minutes every day. But very few people are as active as they should or could be. So how can you motivate your child (and you) to be more active? People do (or do not do) exercise for many reasons. If we understand these reasons, then we can understand how to become more active. Below are the many reasons why people exercise, along with tips for encouraging your child to become more active. These also involve the same strategies as being a good role model, managing the home environment and saying the right things.

'As part of my life'

The main reason for being active is that it is 'just part of my life'. Therefore, if children walk to school, play in the garden, climb trees, cycle to their friend's house or play active games at home (rather than sitting in front of the TV or computer), they will be exercising without knowing it and staying healthy with the minimum amount of effort. Similarly, if adults walk to work or at least use public transport, use stairs rather than lifts, walk up escalators, walk to the shops or out for the evening and keep sitting at home or work to the minimum, they, too, will be doing exercise without having to think about it. To encourage children to be more active, build exercise into your daily life with the children; walk to school if possible; walk to the shops at the weekend or walk around to friends' houses; try to have active weekends and holidays; turn the TV off and throw the children into the garden; limit computer time; be a good role model and be seen to be active; make positive comments about being active, such as, 'Isn't it nice to be outdoors'; 'We have lovely chats when we walk', 'Parking takes such a long time'.

'To be with friends'

The second main reason why people exercise is that it provides social contact. This is why group sports such as football, basketball and netball are popular with children. It is also why adults join gyms to attend dance, aerobic or spinning classes so that they can exercise while being with other people. Exercise is more likely to happen if it is a social activity which brings with it social benefits. In order to help children to be more active encourage lunch time and after school activities; organise with other parents to get your children to do activities together; have friends for tea and throw them all out in the garden; take them to the park with friends when possible; take another family along for weekend walks – the children will stop moaning and run off happily.

'It's fun'

Most exercise campaigns emphasise health benefits and tell people that keeping active is good for their heart, helps them live longer and helps them maintain a healthy weight. None of this means anything to children, who live in the present and find it hard to worry about next week, let alone having a heart attack when they are 65. Even adults do not really think about their health until they have symptoms and find they cannot climb stairs, sit on the floor or run for a bus. And even then, they often just accept this and stop trying. We are very bad at 'future thinking' and are only really concerned with the here and now. Therefore, the next main reason why people exercise is having fun. If exercise is fun, the benefits of doing it NOW easily outweigh the costs, and it works by making the here and now more enjoyable. For children, group sports are, therefore, more fun as they are with friends, but other activities such as trampolining, skipping, dancing, climbing trees or cycling up and down hills are more fun than just running round the park. For adults, anything with other people is fun, but also activities which involve music, are a bit like dancing, can be done whilst driving a simulated motorbike, or provide the opportunity to flirt with sweaty people, all make the here and now more enjoyable. The following should help make children more active: talking about exercise is a fun way. Say, 'Was netball fun at school?', 'Did you enjoy PE today?', 'I used to love skipping when I was your age', and NOT, 'Was it cold in PE today?', 'I used to hate having to play netball', 'Those PE teachers are mean making you go outside'; think of fun and cheap ways to get them active: buy a skipping rope, a ball, even a yoyo is better than sitting around; play music and dance around with them; get them to put on dance shows; clear a space and get them to do gymnastics.

Weighing up the costs and benefits of exercise

Given that we live very much in the moment, at the time of choosing to be active, the benefits at that time need to outweigh the costs. There are, however, many costs that get in the way such as 'it's time consuming', 'it's boring', 'it takes time', 'I'm busy', 'I don't like getting sweaty', 'I don't like having to change', 'it's embarrassing as I'm not very fit' and 'it costs too much to join a gym'. Exercise, therefore, needs to be done in a way that avoids these costs. For example, if your child finds exercise boring, try to find a game they like that is fun – computer games that involve jumping, dancing or pretend fighting are a good way to get them moving without realising it. If your child feels they do not have time, work out how much time they spend watching TV or playing on a computer, point this out and make a deal with them to spend half of this time in the garden playing basketball or join an after-school activity. Also, try to make sure you make it easier for them to be active and harder for them to just sit; turn the TV off, limit computer games and suggest an active alternative; get them to walk to school every day if possible and buy a skipping rope for them or get them a football for the garden. That way, the benefits of doing exercise will outweigh the costs.

Social norms

One key factor that determines whether people exercise is whether being active is the norm in their family or social group. For children, if they have active friends or go to a school where exercise is valued and seen as important, they will become more active. And central to setting this norm are the parents and the family environment. If parents drive everywhere, then children will grow up believing walking is boring and a waste of time. If weekends are spent in front of the TV and holidays are spent lying on a beach, then children will think that this is how their leisure time should be spent. But if parents role model how fun, useful, exciting, and NORMAL exercise is, then children will grow up seeing it as a central part of their lives. So, create positive social norms by being a good role model and being seen to enjoy being active; use the car less and have an active day every weekend. Also encourage friendships with active children and talk about how nice it is to be active, saying, 'I feel so much better after a walk', 'I do love fresh air' and 'You seemed to have such a lovely time playing in the garden with Sophie?' That way, being active will become the norm, and children will carry it through to their adult lives.

Confidence

Feeling confident is also key to being active. This can involve being confident at sports such as swimming, basketball, football or tennis. It can also mean feeling confident that you know where the changing rooms are at the local leisure centre, knowing how to pay to get in, knowing where to get the bus from or knowing the route to walk to school. Children who are not used to doing much will feel that being active is frightening, intimidating and different, which will be a great barrier to becoming more active. The best way to build confidence is simply to do something a few times, congratulate yourself on having done it and then do it more. For your children, you may need to bribe them in the first instance, but bribery is fine if it works and gets them more active. For example, walk with them to school at first, then walk some of the way, then let them walk alone (if it is not too far!); let them go to the leisure centre with their friends; set up a reward system for every time they do something active. This could be simple, such as stickers on a chart, or pasta pieces in a jar. It could be more complex, such as buying a ticket for something they want to go to, making them earn it week by week, or even paying them monthly with pocket money if they achieve the targets you have set. It is bribery, really, but it works, and it is worth it if they are healthier in the long run. And try giving them their pocket money in chunks – some for activities and some for whatever they like.

Habit

We are creatures of habit, and the best predictor of how we will behave in the future is how we have behaved in the past. Therefore, once a child has started to walk to school, although they may complain at first, this will quickly become a habit, and they will stop thinking about it. Similarly, once they have used the stairs a few times when out and about, they will soon realise that this is often quicker and less frustrating than waiting behind someone on the escalators or staring at closed lift doors. You can even make it into a race: you get the lift and see if they can beat you by using the stairs (and always make them win!). Habits are set up early in life and very soon become the norm. Try to do this with exercise so that being active throughout the day feels like the normal way to be. Once established, a habit is very difficult to change.

Planning

Much of our behaviour is spontaneous and in response to triggers or cues throughout the day. This can lead to unhealthy behaviour and the continuation of unhealthy habits. One way to break this pattern is to make clear and explicit plans and to write these down. These then become a kind of contract with yourself and others, and are surprisingly hard to break. Good examples are to plan to walk to school with the children, walk to work or walk into town; or to plan to go for a bike ride at the weekend or to go swimming after school. BUT do not make general plans, such as 'I will walk more' or 'I will be more active'. Make them as specific as possible, write them down and stick them on the fridge. For example, you could write, 'I will walk to school with the kids on Tuesday and Thursday this week'; 'We will go swimming after school this Wednesday'; 'This Saturday, we will go for a bike ride around the local park at 10:30' or 'This Saturday morning, we will all walk into town at 11:00'. Make this list public, tell everyone what you are planning and then tick them off when you have done them. This way, it is far more likely that you will do what you say you are going to do.

Valuing health

For most people, being healthy is not a great motivator as it is too far in the future and the immediate benefits of being unhealthy (eating cake NOW, watching TV NOW) will always outweigh something in 5 or 10, or even 50 years' time. But some degree of valuing health is bound to influence how we behave and how active our children are. Therefore, try to generate a general feeling that it is good to be active and that health **is** important. You do not need to become a nag or a bore to do this, but just point out other people who are being active or inactive and be seen and heard to believe that health is important. For example, point out how healthy their friends are who play sport; talk about TV personalities who are active and good role models; be a good role model yourself and be seen and heard to enjoy being busy, mobile and active; make comments such as, 'Isn't it great to be out of the house', 'How lovely to be in the fresh air', 'I feel so much better after that walk', 'Wasn't swimming fun' and 'We always talk much better when we are out and about'.

Happiness

There is good evidence that exercise is good for our mood. This may take the form of a 'runner's high' for those who are very fit, but for most people, it is just a sense of happiness, being alive, and a release of stress when we are outdoors in the fresh air and being active. Make sure your children start to think of exercise as a way to manage their emotions and give them the clear message that exercise can be an excellent way for them to cope with the stresses of their lives. For example, if they are fed up, take them for a walk around the block or encourage them to play outside for a while; make comments such as, 'go and let off some steam' or 'exercise will make you feel better'; When they seem better, reinforce this and say, 'See that worked, didn't it. Exercise is a great way to get rid of stress'; be a good role model, and when you are fed up, be seen and heard to go for a run or a walk around the block.

In summary

Being active protects against many illnesses, such as heart disease, diabetes, hypertension and obesity, and it also strengthens bones and muscles. It also has psychological benefits and improves body confidence, wellbeing and reduces depression and anxiety. In the main, people do exercise because it is part of their weekly routine, it is fun, and they can do it with other people. Children can be encouraged to be more active by addressing these factors by building it into their daily routines and making it both fun and sociable.

To conclude

Children often go through stages of not liking how they look and can feel that they are too fat, too thin, too tall or too short or just a bit spotty. This can lead to poor self-esteem and lower their mood. As a parent, it is important to listen and acknowledge their feelings whilst also building up their self-esteem and creating a sense that we are much more than just how we look. This can be achieved through being a good role model for body image and keeping quiet about any of your own body issues, saying the right things by talking about people positively and not focusing on how they look and managing the home environment through getting rid of the bathroom scales and removing any bedroom mirrors. Children can also become very sedentary, particularly in their teenage years. This chapter has also highlighted how you can encourage them to be more active again by focusing on the more immediate benefits of exercise, such as having fun and being with friends and using the pillars of good parenting.

REFERENCE

1. Ogden, J. (2024). The inews. I wish I'd told my children they were beautiful.   https://inews.co.uk/inews-lifestyle/psychologist-wish-told-children-beautiful-2941099

SECTION III

ADULTHOOD – HAVING A GOOD RELATIONSHIP WITH FOOD

6

WHY IS LOSING
WEIGHT SO HARD?

What and how we eat as adults relates to our childhoods and how we were food-parented by our own parents. It also relates to the people we spend our time with as adults, as we can change our diets to fit in with our friends or partners, and even our own children. Our diets are also very much influenced by our environments and the kinds of food we are surrounded by at work, in cafés and restaurants and the shops we visit. This can often result in overeating and subsequent weight gain. This first chapter in the adult section of this book will explore why we overeat, with a focus on what is in our heads and the impact of the food environment. It will then describe why people diet and the physical and psychological consequences of trying to eat less. Finally, it will explore why it is so hard to eat less and how trying to eat less can be undermined by factors such as emotional triggers, withdrawal, scripts, cross addiction, physical triggers and social pressure.

WHY DO WE OVEREAT?

The energy in/energy out equation is a very fine balance, and even just eating one extra piece of toast per day that you do not need can result in weight gain after a year. Imagine how quickly this could turn

DOI: 10.4324/9781003600183-11

into becoming overweight or developing obesity! It is clear, therefore, that people who are overweight have eaten more than they needed in the past. It is also clear that to maintain this level of weight, they must be eating exactly what they need; otherwise, their weight would go down. Weight maintenance is hard. Weight loss is even harder. When asked why they eat, most people say, 'I'm hungry' or 'I like it', and they tend to see eating behaviour as a biological need driven by the need to survive. Eating behaviour is much more complex than this, as we eat for so many reasons other than hunger: 'I was bored', I was unhappy', 'It was there', 'I needed to clear my plate', 'Sunday lunch is a big family time', 'I was out with my friends'. At its simplest, eating can be seen as the result of what is in our heads and the triggers in our environment, which, in turn, can lead to overeating.

How are we impacted by what is in our heads?

From the moment we are born, we learn to like certain foods in the same way that we learn to speak, to like certain clothes or to enjoy certain hobbies (see Chapter 2). We learn through exposure and simply prefer the foods we are more familiar with. We learn by watching our parents, peers or the media and by seeing foods that others eat, particularly if those people are the ones we love or want to be like. And we learn through the simple process of reward and association. So, if our parents said, 'Eat your vegetables and you can have pudding', 'You have been good, have a piece of cake', 'Have you had a difficult day? Have a biscuit', or 'Let's have a treat and go out for ice cream', we learn that sweet foods are treats and vegetables are boring, and that treat foods make us feel special and are a great way to manage our emotions. And this leaves us with a set of schemas in our heads, which we carry through into adulthood and use to determine what foods we like, when we eat and how much we eat. These are the factors that cause overeating, which can be seen in terms of the following factors.

Emotional eating

When a child is upset, the easiest and quickest way to calm them down is to give them food. This acts as a distraction from the feelings they are having; it gives them something to do with their hands and mouth and shifts their attention from whatever was upsetting them. If the food chosen is also seen as a treat, such as sweets or a biscuit, then the child will feel 'treated' and happier. In the short term, using food like this is effective. But in the long term, it can be harmful as we quickly learn that food is a good way to manage emotions. Then, as we go through life, whenever we feel fed up, anxious or even just bored, we turn to food to make ourselves feel better. This is known as emotional eating, and studies indicate that emotional eating is linked with weight gain (1,2).

Social interaction

Food should be about hunger and fullness and seen as a simple fuel to keep the body going. Yet, because of the way food is used in families and society in general, we develop a wide range of associations between food and other aspects of our lives. One of the key associations is between food and social interactions, and so for many people, food is not only about managing emotions but also about family time, birthdays, weddings, religious festivals, dating and the celebration of just about any occasion that involves being with other people. And for many, this leads to overeating and subsequent weight gain.

Identity

Food also plays a central role in the way that we see ourselves and forms a core part of our identity. People, therefore, may see themselves as picky eaters, fussy or choosy about what they eat, whilst others declare 'I eat anything'. Some become very health-conscious and will only eat low-fat, low-sugar, low-salt diets and turn to avoiding meat, additives and processed foods, whilst others announce that nutritionists cannot make their minds up about what we should eat and 'it's all nonsense' and, therefore, pride themselves in eating everything. And whilst some publicly proclaim, 'I don't have much of an appetite these days', others proudly say, 'I can eat like a horse'. These are all ways of using food as part of how we see ourselves and how we communicate who we are to the world around us. Food becomes a language to speak with and can result in eating more than we need and becoming overweight.

Guilt and denial

For some, food is a pleasure and a treat and part of the way in which they feel better about life. But for many, food is also linked with guilt and negativity. There is so much pressure to be thin, with all its associations of attractiveness, control and emotional stability, that people deny themselves food to lose weight. But then, as this process of denial can only last so long, they end up eating and swing between eating, guilt about eating and subsequent overeating to manage the guilt. This, in turn, can lead to weight gain.

Food and reward

Food is linked to reward in many ways. Eating food is rewarding as it tastes nice and makes us feel good. Food is also used as a reward when we deserve a treat, take a break from work or have met one of our goals. And food can also be used as a reward for eating or not eating food, as in: 'I have finished my dinner, so I can have my pudding' or 'I have stuck to my diet and so deserve a piece of cake'. As a result, unhealthy food often takes on the meaning of 'treat' whilst healthy food is seen as boring or just necessary. The problem with weight gain is that all these rewards are in the here and now, whereas the negative consequences of weight gain are always in the future. And people do 'future discounting' and so the benefits and rewards now always beat the costs in the future; cake now always beats a heart attack in 40 years, and so we overeat, and our weight goes up (3).

A simple cost-benefit analysis

At its simplest, eating behaviour is really a cost-benefit analysis with people weighing up the benefits (managing emotions, being sociable, making a statement about identity, pleasure and reward) against the costs (guilt, risk, obesity, diabetes and heart disease). Unfortunately, when it comes to food, most of the benefits are in the here and now, and most of the costs are in the future, which means that the benefits mostly win, and people end up eating more than they should.

Eating is, therefore, a response to how we think about food and 'what is in our heads'. Eating is also a response to triggers in our environment.

How are we influenced by triggers in the environment?

The obesogenic environment makes it very easy to eat and offers a wide range of triggers which cause mindless eating and change what, when, where, how and why we eat.

What we eat

Bags of crisps used to be 30 g, and we would eat these and stop. Many bags are now 'grab bags' and are 60 g. Very few people eat the original 30g and then stop; they eat the lot – twice the amount they used to eat. We now live in a world where portion sizes are bigger, cakes are offered around at work, we have snacks in our cupboards and 'drive-in' fast food restaurants where we can buy thousands of calories' worth of food without even having to stop driving to eat it. And we eat it not because we are hungrier than we used to be, but because it is there. And when we are eating it, we do so without realising that we are eating, and as a result, it does not make us full. This is known as mindless eating (4). We did a study looking at how much people ate in four different situations: in the car, watching TV, chatting to someone or on their own. We found two results (5). First, people ate more whilst watching TV than in any of the other situations, which has also been found in many other studies (e.g. 6). Second, the amount they ate whilst driving was unrelated to changes in their hunger. This indicates that we eat more when we are distracted, particularly when watching TV. It also indicates that if we are distracted, as when we are driving, we do not register the food we have eaten, and it does not make us full. In turn, this has also been shown to lead to even more eating later (7). Such mindless eating makes people overeat in an environment where food is easily available, and over time, this causes weight gain. The environment, therefore, changes what we eat, and we can end up mindlessly eating more food than tends to be higher in calories.

When we eat

The obesogenic environment also means that we are far more likely to eat snacks than meals, and unfortunately, snacks are often higher in fat and calories and more likely to be forgotten or discounted. If you ask someone what they ate yesterday, they will tell you their breakfast, lunch and dinner, but not the snacks (or drinks) in between. This means that snacking makes people eat more in the long term, as they have not registered that they have eaten and therefore do not feel as full. There is also some evidence that those who are overweight may be more likely to skip meals, particularly breakfast, which may make them more likely to snack throughout the rest of the day (8).

Where we eat

There have also been changes to where people eat, and not only do people eat more snacks, but they also eat these snacks on the go, either in the car, at their desks or in the street. We did a study of the impact of 'eating on the go' and found that those who ate a cereal bar whilst walking around the corridors of the university consumed more later than those who ate the cereal bar sitting down at a table. Eating on the go seemed to make people feel less full afterwards, meaning that they carried on eating when food was made available again (9). And then, when people do sit down to eat, they often eat in front of the TV, which can also increase food intake (5). This is because they are distracted from eating and so do not notice how much they have consumed.

How we eat

Weight gain may also be related to how we eat, with heavier people tending to show a faster initial rate of eating and to take larger spoonfuls of food (10). This may be because they are eating food as snacks, eating on the go rather than as a meal or due to higher levels of emotional eating, which makes them anxious around food.

Why we eat

Ideally, we would eat when we are hungry and stop when we are full. But as described above, we eat for many other reasons, as food is used as a way to manage our emotions, for social interaction, to make statements of our identity, and all the factors that are in our heads. The environment around us not only changes when, where, what and how we eat; it also changes why we eat, and it also acts as a trigger for these different reasons. If food is there, we eat mindlessly, rather than when we are hungry. But if the environment triggers our emotions, we eat for emotional regulation; if we are in a café, we eat for social interaction; if we are with certain people in our lives, we eat to make a statement about how we want these people to see us.

In summary

At its simplest, weight gain is a result of us eating more than we need. This chapter has explored the reasons why people overeat, with a focus on what is in our heads and the triggers in our environment. It has also been shown that, at times, these triggers in our environment then change which part of what is in our heads is most important. And this can all lead to weight gain. As a result, people then try to lose weight through dieting. This is only sometimes successful.

WHY DO PEOPLE DIET, AND WHAT ARE THE CONSEQUENCES?

Dieting comes in many forms and has positive and negative consequences for the dieter. This section will describe what dieting is and when people diet. It will then explore the impact of dieting on physical factors such as weight, health status and mortality and psychological factors such as mood, eating behaviour and identity.

What is dieting?

Since about the 1960s, there has been an endless stream of new diets on the market, including those recommending eating only fruit, only meat or only meal substitute drinks; those excluding whole food groups such as carbohydrates, fats, protein or sugars; and those recommending missing meals, calorie counting, a points system, having days on and days off or following a healthy eating meal plan. A recent study synthesised 72 research projects and identified 37 weight loss strategies, the most common being eating more fruit and vegetables, selecting food more consciously, eating soup and self-weighing (11). The researchers also identified 12 motivations, of which the most common were to improve well-being, to improve health and prevent disease and to improve fitness and appearance.

But whatever the method, at its essence, a diet is anything that suggests that you eat less than you usually would and impose some level of control over your eating to lose weight. This study also explored the prevalence of dieting and indicated that about 42% of the general population report trying to lose weight in the past year, about 23% report trying to maintain weight loss in the past year, and about 70% report having ever dieted to lose weight (11). There are several reasons why people diet, which will now be addressed.

Why do people diet?

Most people diet to try to lose weight for three reasons. First, those who are overweight or living with obesity often diet to lose weight. For some, this involves joining a formal weight management group either via a referral from their doctor or simply by attending on their own. For many, however, it involves self-imposed limits which may be guided through diet books, the internet, apps or self-help groups. Next, although many people diet as a means to improve their health, the more immediate goal is often to improve their body satisfaction. And whilst some with body dissatisfaction may be overweight, many are not but are critical of the way they look. Body dissatisfaction can also be a key driver of dieting behaviour, but it is not always a healthy one. Third, dieting is also at the heart of eating disorders and can be very problematic. There are many different eating disorders (EDs), including anorexia nervosa (AN; excessive weight loss), bulimia nervosa (BN; bingeing and purging), binge eating disorder (BED; binge eating but without purging), orthorexia (excessive concern about healthy eating) and eating disorder not otherwise specified (EDNOS), a general term for other forms of ED which do not quite fulfil the criteria for other problems (see Chapter 1). These all involve some form of food restriction and dieting.

People, therefore, diet for many reasons. All these approaches to dieting have implications for physical and psychological health and well-being.

How does dieting impact our physical health?

Dieting changes our physical health in a number of ways.

Weight loss

If effective, dieting can lead to weight loss, and evidence indicates that about 60% of people who diet lose weight in the first six months. This is increased to about 70% with some form of sustained follow-up from a health professional. A review of the evidence by NICE, however, indicated that by one year, those who had received best-case behavioural management from either public sector or private sector weight management behaviour change services, such as the NHS, Weight Watchers or Slimming World, showed an average weight loss of 2.22 kg (12). Similarly, a review of those interventions focusing on food intake and physical activity showed an average of 1.56 kg less weight regain by one year compared to controls (13). Further, a trial of those referred to a commercial weight loss company through the NHS indicated that whilst two-thirds lost less than 5% of their body weight, one-third lost more than 5% after at least starting a 12-week course (14). There is always variation around these figures; however, with some people losing more weight and some losing less.

Health status

Although weight losses can seem small following dieting attempts, evidence indicates that when people are overweight, even 10% weight loss causes a dramatic reduction in the risk of heart disease and stroke, a reversal of Type 2 diabetes so that a person can start to regulate their own blood sugars again and a reduction in the risk of weight-related cancers such as breast cancer and endometrial cancer in women (15). Further, weight loss of more than 10% can bring even greater health benefits (16). Being overweight is also strongly linked to shorter life expectancy (17). Losing weight can improve life expectancy if this weight loss is sustained. Furthermore, regardless of mortality and more serious health conditions, weight loss can also improve a person's daily physical health through the reduction of symptoms such as breathlessness, back and knee pain and the susceptibility to minor infections.

Yo-yo dieting and weight regain

Unfortunately, although most people who diet manage to lose weight initially, many show weight regain by a five-year follow-up. Some research suggests that having some periods of time in your life when you weigh less, even if this weight is regained, may be healthier in the same way that stopping smoking for the odd month or even year gives the lungs time to recover (18). Other research indicates, however, that yo-yo dieting (i.e. showing large fluctuations in weight) may be harmful, even more harmful than remaining at a more stable higher weight (19). This is because when a person loses weight, they often lose muscle and fat, but when they put it back on, they regain proportionally more fat, making them not only heavier but fatter over time. In turn, this has a negative impact on their cardiovascular health, can add to fatty liver disease and exacerbates their risk of diabetes. It would be a shame if this deterred people from trying to lose weight, but it does indicate the negative side of failed dieting.

How does dieting impact our psychological health?

Dieting also has many psychological consequences, and again, this often depends on whether dieting leads to weight loss and whether this weight loss is sustained.

Mood, confidence and body image

Weight loss can lead to improved mood and a reduction in anxiety and depression. Those who lose weight also report increases in self-confidence and body image, although this can sometimes take time as people need to internalise their new body size and sometimes report buying clothes that are too large whilst they learn to come to terms with their body shape. When weight is regained, however, these improvements are seldom sustained, with people sometimes reporting feeling worse than before as they see themselves as having failed and let themselves down.

Identity

When dieting is successful, many people describe a sense of being 'reborn', of having 'a second chance', or being a 'new person' and feeling 'liberated'. This shift in identity can result in a change of job, a new relationship or a determination to live life to the fullest. It sometimes also leads to people becoming spokespersons for weight loss, setting up their own dieting company or becoming very passionate about exercise and healthy eating. Interestingly, those who show such a shift in their identity also seem more likely to keep their weight off in the longer term as they have more invested in success (20).

Preoccupation with food

At its heart, dieting involves not eating food that people want to eat, and whether this involves avoiding whole food groups, eating fewer calories or just eating less, it always involves some level of denial. As a result, many dieters develop a preoccupation with the very thing they are trying not to have – food. This has been called a paradoxical effect, as trying not to think about something makes people think about it more and is exactly what happens to a lot of people when they diet. For the majority, the preoccupation with food takes the form of thinking about food for a disproportionate amount of time. For others, this can become more pathological, leading to eating disorders, such as AN or BN.

Overeating

At times, dieting can result in people eating less and losing weight. But for many, trying to eat less often results in people eating more. This may be in the form of compensatory overeating when people simply eat the amount or types of foods they have been avoiding. At times, however, this can also result in binge eating. This has been called the 'what the hell' effect and occurs when people feel that they have broken their diet through eating a food that was not allowed, when they have a low mood and overeat to cheer themselves up, or after drinking alcohol, when their resistance is lowered. Such overeating can then make people feel worse about themselves, which in turn can lower self-esteem and trigger guilt, which may lead to further overeating as people use food to manage their emotions.

In summary

Dieting involves trying to eat less as a means to lose weight and can be a response to being overweight or obese, body dissatisfaction or even an ED. Dieting has implications for both physical and psychological health, and when it is effective, people show improvements in their risks for diseases such as heart disease and diabetes and a reduction in symptoms such as breathlessness and joint pain. They can also experience improved mood and body satisfaction. At times, dieting can lead to weight loss followed by weight regain, which may be worse for health than just remaining overweight. It can also trigger a preoccupation with food and overeating.

WHY IS IT SO HARD TO EAT LESS?

Much of our eating behaviours are habits created as a result of modelling, repetition, reinforcement and association (see Chapter 2). Changing eating behaviour is, therefore, difficult as it involves breaking these habits. Many diets fail because, as much as we might want to eat less and change what and when we eat, this is often undermined by what is in our head, such as emotional triggers, withdrawal, scripts, cross-addiction and factors in the environment, such as physical triggers and social pressure.

How are we undermined by what is in our heads?

There are many factors inside our heads that make it very hard to eat less.

Emotional triggers

Eating behaviour is often the result of certain triggers, and every time we come across these triggers, we are prompted to behave in a particular way. Some of these triggers are in our heads, such as our mood (e.g. feeling fed up) and are, therefore, very difficult to avoid as they follow us everywhere and are hard to ignore. And because eating habits often require so little thought, much of the time we are not even aware of what we are doing or how our emotions are determining what foods we eat.

Withdrawal and feelings of worry and stress

Habits are part of our everyday lives, and therefore, when we do not clean our teeth, eat breakfast, have our morning coffee or have biscuits in the afternoon, we feel unsettled and a little bit stressed.

This feeling is unpleasant, and we quickly learn that it can be avoided by carrying on with our habit. Therefore, not eating biscuits feels unusual, but this can all be made OK with a few biscuits. And the habit carries on as it becomes the solution to the problem created when trying to change it. It is a vicious circle. But it is the change in the habit which makes us feel stressed, not the absence of the actual behaviour. And if we start to realise that the feeling of stress or worry is just 'withdrawal' and will only be made worse in the longer term if we give in and use the habit to get rid of it, then we can start to break the habit itself.

Scripts in our heads

From an early age, we develop scripts in our heads of what we like and do not like, who we are and what we do. These scripts come from the people around us, particularly our parents, and tell us whether we are a good or bad person. For example, some people have negative scripts in their heads which say, 'I am always late', 'I'm a problem', 'I'm selfish', 'I never try my best' or 'I'm stupid'. Other people may have more positive scripts which tell them 'I am kind', 'I am thoughtful', 'I work hard', 'I always stick at things' and 'I'm clever'. In terms of eating habits, these scripts can make it very difficult to change if we tell ourselves, 'I have a problem with food', 'Eating is my only crutch in life' or 'I have an addictive personality'. Although some of these scripts may feel 'true' and reflect how people behave, they make it more difficult to change, as breaking a long-standing habit not only means changing the behaviour but also changing the very way in which a person sees themselves. And this is hard.

Denial and rebound effects

When people try to change their habits, they are mostly attempting to stop doing something they still want to do. So, people on a diet may like crisps but try not to eat them, and those trying to be active would rather read a book but try to get to an exercise class. This makes changing behaviour difficult because it always introduces an element of denial, and human beings are hopeless at denying themselves something if they want it and it is available. Furthermore, the process of denial makes the behaviour we are trying to deny ourselves even more attractive and desirable than it was before, which can create rebound effects. So, if we say to ourselves, 'Today, I will not eat cake', automatically, we think about cake more, not less. Then, because we are thinking about cake more but cannot have it, we want it more as the day progresses. Eventually, when we give in and have cake, not only do we now want it more than we did in the morning, but we also end up eating more cake because we have been denying ourselves all day. This is a very powerful effect, which means that by making food forbidden and putting ourselves into denial, we paradoxically become more preoccupied with food, and when we do give in (which most people do), we paradoxically eat more than if we had not denied ourselves in the first place. This is called the 'what the hell' effect.

A challenged identity

Although people who are overweight may not like being overweight and want to be thinner, their identity can often be tied up with their body size. When they first start to lose weight, this can be rewarding as they may feel healthier and can see their body shape changing. But with this comes a challenge to their identity as they will feel pressure from themselves and others to be someone different. At this point, some people 'sabotage' their diets as the new thinner version of themselves can be perceived as a threat. This can lead to overeating and weight regain.

Beliefs about food preferences

Food preferences are learned from the moment we are born through exposure to different foods, learning by modelling and watching others and the association between different foods and certain places and feelings. Our food preferences are therefore embedded and feel as if they are fixed in a pattern on our tongues. Dieting can involve eating less of the foods we usually eat. But sometimes, it may involve trying new foods, which can be a challenge to our beliefs about the food we like or dislike. So, if we snack on chocolate or cake in the afternoon, dieting may just involve cutting this out. And if we eat large portions of spaghetti bolognese for our dinner, then a diet would involve a smaller portion. But a diet may also involve finding a substitute for the chocolate or cake, such as fruit, and if we eat lots of chips, then a diet might involve eating rice or boiled potatoes instead. Yet, if we believe that we do not like these foods, then the diet will be hard to follow. And the new, healthier habits will be harder to set up.

Cross addiction

Many people use food to regulate their emotions, and when they are dieting, they need to find an alternative source of support. Ideally, this would be through exercise, talking to friends, going to the cinema or reading a book. But some people need to have a more substantial substitute, and this can lead to cross addiction with some people turning to smoking, alcoholism, shopping or sex addiction. In terms of weight loss, some of these are probably quite useful, but alcohol contains large amounts of hidden calories and can undermine dieting attempts, causing weight regain. It may also lead to the 'what the hell' effect if people become disinhibited and, therefore, overeat.

Eating habits are, therefore, hard to change due to factors inside our heads. Such a change is also hindered by triggers in the environment.

How are we undermined by triggers in the environment?

Eating becomes associated with many different aspects of our environment, which can prompt eating even when we are trying to eat less.

Physical triggers

Some environmental triggers are physical, such as the biscuit tin, the fridge, carefully placed snack foods in supermarkets or the cake trolley at work, which cause mindless shopping and mindless eating. Yet, as with emotional triggers, much of this habitual behaviour is done without thinking; those who overeat and eat biscuits with their afternoon cup of tea do so as this feels normal and not doing so does not feel quite right. Such physical triggers, however, unlike emotional triggers, can be avoided if we make small changes to our daily routines or change our environment.

Social pressure

Our behaviours are intricately linked with other people, and are often central to how we build up our relationships. We may have a friend at work with whom we have cake in the afternoon, a husband who likes to buy us chocolates as a treat or children whom we enjoy taking out for ice cream. If we then try to change our behaviour, these other people in our lives may object, and the pressure is on to behave the way we always have done. Husbands will feel rejected if we do not eat the chocolates, our friend will feel lonely eating cake on their own, we will miss out on the gossip, and ice cream will seem less of a treat. People like us to carry on the way we always have, as it makes them feel safe. If we change, then they feel that they have to change as well, and that is unsettling. This social pressure always increases to maintain the status quo whenever anyone tries to break a habit. This can be through kindness.

Negative social support

Sometimes, this social pressure can be more negative than just being nudged into eating more. We have carried out work exploring negative support and have identified three different types: sabotage, being a feeder and collusion. Sabotage is defined as the 'active and intentional undermining of another person's weight goals', feeding behaviour has been defined as 'explicit over feeding of someone when they are not hungry or wishing not to eat', and collusion has been defined as 'passive and benign negative social support to avoid conflict'. For example, refusing to drive a partner to the gym would be a form of sabotage, and buying someone chocolates when they are trying to eat well would be being a feeder. In contrast, if someone says, 'I can't be bothered to cook, let's get a takeaway' and their partner says, 'Great idea, I'll get a curry', this would be collusion. A better partner would say, 'That's fine, I'll cook tonight' (21–24). Forms of negative social support can be key to how relationships function, and even though they might be motivated from a good place and the desire to keep the relationship the same as it has always been, they can make it very hard to change what we eat. They are a form of 'killing with kindness' and function to maintain the status quo of a relationship, whilst also preventing one part of that relationship from becoming healthier. They can also sometimes be less kind and more malign.

In summary

Habits are a product of modelling, repetition, reinforcement and association and are difficult to change because they have often been entrenched for a very long time. This means that diets often fail as people are unable to change their eating habits. In addition, changing eating habits is made even more difficult due to factors such as emotional triggers, denial and withdrawal and environmental triggers which prompt mindless eating or social pressure from others who want us to carry on as usual.

To conclude

This chapter has explored why people eat more than they need, highlighting the role of what is in our heads and the triggers in the environment. Overeating can lead to weight gain, and at times, people try to diet to lose weight. This can lead to dieting, which has both positive and negative consequences for our physical and mental health. The chapter has also explored why it is so hard to eat less and lose weight, and why so many diets fail, focusing on the role of both internal and external factors. At its simplest, eating behaviours illustrate a simple cost-benefit analysis, and at the time of carrying out the behaviour, the immediate benefits will mostly outweigh the longer-term costs. But sometimes, eating behaviours can be changed. This is addressed in the next chapter in terms of eating less for weight loss and changing eating behaviour for health in general, such as eating more fruit and vegetables, cooking more, eating less meat and avoiding ultra-processed foods.

REFERENCES

1. Koenders, P.G., and van Strien, T. (2011). Emotional eating, rather than lifestyle behavior, drives weight gain in a prospective study in 1562 employees. *Journal of Occupational and Environmental Medicine*, 53, 1287–1293.
2. Konttinen, H., Silventoinen, K., Sarlio-Lähteenkorva, S., Männistö, S., and Haukkala, A. (2010). Emotional eating and physical activity self-efficacy as pathways in the association between depressive symptoms and adiposity indicators. *American Journal of Clinical Nutrition*, 92, 1031–1039.
3. Hall, P.A., and Fong, G.T. (2007). Temporal self-regulation theory: A model for individual health behaviour. *Health Psychology Review*, 1(1), 6–52.
4. Wansink, B. (2009). *Mindless Eating: Why We Eat More than We Think*, 2nd ed. London: Hay House.
5. Ogden, J., Coop, N., Cousins, C., Crump, R., Field, L., Hughes, S., and Woodger, N. (2013). Distraction, the desire to eat and food intake: Towards an expanded model of mindless eating. *Appetite*, 62, 119–126.
6. Bellissimo, N., Pencharz, P.B., Thomas, S.G., and Anderson, G.H. (2007). Effect of television viewing at mealtime on food intake after a glucose preload in boys. *Pediatric Research*, 61(6), 745–749.
7. Higgs, S., and Woodward, M. (2009). Television watching during lunch increases afternoon snack intake of young women. *Appetite*, 52(1), 39–43.

8. Alsharairi, N.A., and Somerset, S.M. (2016). Skipping breakfast in early childhood and its associations with maternal and child BMI: A study of 2–5-year-old Australian children. *European Journal of Clinical Nutrition*, 70(4), 450–455.

9. Ogden, J., Oikonoumou, E., and Alemany, G. (2016). Distraction, restrained eating and disinhibition: An experimental study of food intake and the impact of 'eating on the go.' *International Journal of Health Psychology*, 22(1), 39–50. doi:10.1177/1359105315595119

10. Laessle, R.G., Lehrke, S., and Dückers, S. (2007). Laboratory eating behavior in obesity. *Appetite*, 49, 399–404.

11. Santos, I., Sniehotta, F.F., Marques, M.M., Carraça, E.V., and Teixeira, P.J. (2017). Prevalence of personal weight control attempts in adults: A systematic review and meta-analysis. *Obesity Reviews*, 18(1), 32–50.

12. Hartmann-Boyce, J., Johns, D.J., Jebb, S.A., Summerbell, C., and Aveyard, P. (2014). Behavioural weight management review group: Behavioural weight management programmes for adults assessed by trials conducted in everyday contexts: Systematic review and meta-analysis. *Obesity Reviews*, 15(11), 920–932.

13. Dombrowski, S.U., Knittle, K., Avenell, A., Araújo-Soares, V., and Sniehotta, F.F. (2014). Long term maintenance of weight loss with non-surgical interventions in obese adults: Systematic review and meta-analyses of randomised controlled trials. *BMJ*, 14, 348.

14. Ahern, A.L., Olson, A.D., Aston, L.M., and Jebb, S.A. (2011). Weight Watchers on prescription: An observational study of weight change among adults referred to Weight Watchers by the NHS. *BMC Public Health*, 11, 434.

15. Warkentin, L.M., Majumdar, S.R., Johnson, J.A., et al. (2014). Weight loss required by the severely obese to achieve clinically important differences in health-related quality of life: two-year prospective cohort study. *BMC Medicine*, 12, 175. doi:10.1186/s12916-014-0175-5

16. Tahrani, A.A., and Morton, J. (2022). Benefits of weight loss of 10% or more in patients with overweight or obesity: A review. *Obesity (Silver Spring, Md.)*, 30(4), 802–840. https://doi.org/10.1002/oby.23371

17. Ortega, F.B., Cadenas-Sanchez, C., Migueles, J.H., Labayen, I., Ruiz, J.R., Sui, X., Blair, S.N., Martínez-Vizcaino, V., and Lavie, C.J. (2018). Role of physical activity and fitness in the characterization and prognosis of the metabolically healthy obesity phenotype: A systematic review and meta-analysis. *Progress in Cardiovascular Diseases*, 61(2), 190–205. https://doi.org/10.1016/j.pcad.2018.07.008

18. Blackburn, G. (1995). Effect of degree of weight loss on health benefits. *Obesity Reviews*, 3(Supplement 2), 211s–216s.

19. Lissner, L., Odell, P.M., D'Agostino, R.B., Stokes, J., Kreger, B.E., Belanger, A.J., and Brownell, K.D. (1991). Variability of body weight and health outcomes in the Framingham population. *New England Journal of Medicine*, 324, 1839–1844.

20. Epiphaniou, E., and Ogden, J. (2010). Successful weight loss maintenance: From a restricted to liberated self. *International Journal of Health Psychology*, 15, 887–896.

21. Ogden, J., and Quirke-McFarlane, S. (2023). Sabotage, collusion and being a feeder: towards a new model of negative social support and its impact on weight management. *Current Obesity Reports*, https://doi.org/10.1007/s13679-023-00504-5

22. Quirke-McFarlane, S., and Ogden, J. (2024). Care or sabotage? A reflexive thematic analysis of perceived partner support throughout the bariatric surgery journey. *British Journal of Health Psychology* 29, 835–854, doi: 10.1111/bjhp.12733

23. Quirke-McFarlane S, and Ogden J. (2024). Is anyone else's husband trying to undermine them all the time?: A reflexive thematic analysis of online support forum discussions about bariatric surgery saboteurs. *Journal of Health Psychology*, 0(0). doi:10.1177/13591053241305946

24. Stiefel F., Michaud, L., Bourquin-Sachse, C., Quirke-McFarlane S., Ogden, J. (2025). Sabotage, feeding and collusion after bariatric surgery. And the winner is . . .? A psychodynamic and systemic perspective on sabotage and feeding after bariatric surgery by means of a case series analysis. *Health*, 0(0). doi:10.1177/13634593251319928

7

HOW CAN I CHANGE
WHAT I EAT?

People want to change their diets in many ways, including eating more fruit and vegetables, cutting back on ultra-processed foods, cooking more and eating fewer takeaways or cutting out meat. Most commonly, though, people want to eat less to lose weight. This chapter will first examine the research evidence from both quantitative research and people's own stories, which highlight a role for factors such as an initial trigger, the belief that things can change, a shift in the cost-benefit analysis for eating and exercise, a new behaviour regimen, a sense of control and a new identity. It then uses this evidence to describe how these factors can be incorporated into an individual's own attempts at behaviour change for weight loss. Weight loss, however, is not the only goal of dietary change. This chapter will then end by outlining the lessons learned from existing research on weight loss to explore how to change your daily diet in other ways, such as eating more fruit and vegetables, snacking less, eating less meat or cutting down on ultra-processed foods. In essence, this involves choosing the right time to change, believing that things can change, shifting the costs/benefits analysis, creating a new behaviour regimen and embedding all these changes into a new sense of self that becomes part of who you are. Together, these processes help to

DOI: 10.4324/9781003600183-12

avoid any rebound effects and make new habits more likely to be sustained in the longer term.

HOW DO PEOPLE MANAGE TO CHANGE THEIR DIET TO LOSE WEIGHT?

Although dieting is hard, some people do manage to eat less and lose weight. Some people also manage to sustain this weight loss. Research has taken different approaches to explore why some people manage to lose weight and keep it off.

What does the research say?

Some studies have compared those who have been successful in losing weight in the long term to those who have been less successful. For example, using the National Weight Control Registry (NWCR) in the US, which is a database established in 1993, researchers concluded that weight loss maintenance over 5 years was related to increased physical activity, decreased intake of fat, increased dietary restraint (i.e. more dieting efforts), having a significant medical trigger and maintaining a consistent diet regimen across the week rather than a more flexible approach to dieting (1). In a similar vein, I concluded from my study (2) that compared to those who had not lost weight, weight loss maintainers tended to be older, had dieted for longer, were lighter at the start, reported higher levels of healthy eating (not calorie counting) and showed a lower endorsement of a medical cause of their weight problem (i.e. not genetic), a stronger endorsement of the psychological consequences of being overweight (e.g. body image) and stated that they were motivated to lose weight for psychological reasons (e.g. self-esteem and confidence). Furthermore, a review of the literature (3) concluded that successful weight loss and maintenance was related to greater initial weight loss, reaching a self-determined weight goal, being physically active, eating regular meals throughout the day including breakfast, healthy eating, showing control of overeating, self-monitoring of behaviour, being motivated by internal reasons, good coping strategies and a sense of control, autonomy and responsibility. Finally, a study by myself and my colleague (4) directly tested some of the factors identified by our research on success stories and concluded that those who sustained the weight they had lost reported a greater incidence of life events, a belief in the psychological (not medical) solutions to their weight problem and a sense of the new healthier behaviours having more benefits than the older unhealthy behaviours.

Other quantitative studies have taken the data from large-scale interventions to explore what factors predict weight loss maintenance in the longer term. For example, research again using the National Weight Control Registry (NWCR) found that larger weight losses and a longer duration of weight loss maintenance were related to increased physical activity in maintainers' leisure time, higher levels of dietary restraint, increased self-weighing, decreased intake of fat and a reduced number of episodes of overeating (5). Further, one study pooled data across a number of studies and highlighted that successful dieting was associated with having a higher baseline weight, being male, showing early weight loss when part of an intervention, attendance at the weight loss intervention, increased length of treatment, increased social support, self-monitoring of behaviours, goal setting, slowing rate of eating and increased physical activity (6). Finally, a comprehensive analysis (7) explored the predictors of weight loss by 12 months and reported key roles for calorie counting, greater contact with a dietician and the use of strategies which involved comparison with others.

These two approaches to understanding sustained weight loss have clearly identified some overlapping variables and suggest a pattern of factors relating to success. In particular, it seems that being male, older, losing more weight at the start, keeping on trying, believing that behaviour is important and that it is not all down to genetics, doing more activity and greater input from health professionals all seem to help.

What do people say?

To provide greater insight into how and why some people manage to change their eating behaviour and eat less, the next approach has been to ask people who have lost weight and kept it off for their own personal stories. This approach has identified a number of factors relating to sustained changes in eating behaviour and subsequent weight loss (8–13).

Being triggered by a life event

Successful weight loss and weight loss maintenance often seem to happen after people have had a life event of some sort. People have called these events many things, such as 'seeing the light', 'an epiphany', 'reaching rock bottom', 'a tipping point' or just a time when the normal pattern of life is shaken up and habits can be broken more easily. For some, this could be a relationship breakdown, a change of job, moving house, reaching a salient milestone such as having a significant birthday, or simply going on holiday. For example, one woman described how the break-up of her marriage had offered her the opportunity to lose weight:

> I just had to take stock of my life … I have gone through a break-up of a marriage, but I have still got two children … It's just something inside you that says if you don't sort yourself out. I think losing weight was the hardest and biggest thing that I have achieved.

(Jackie)

For some, it could be feeling breathless when going up stairs or being diagnosed with a health condition. One man described a very serious version of a health crisis:

> I suppose it was like a new life for me … when you know you are going to die and when I did get up from the coma … I think it was the first time in my life that I really, really did want to lose the weight …

(Tanvir)

Specific events, therefore, seem to make it easier to change how we eat and lose weight. In part, this is because they can shake up the pattern of our lives. It is also, however, because they offer up an opportunity to reinvent who we are and redefine ourselves in better and healthier ways.

It cannot just be the life event itself, however, but the ways in which it makes us think about our lives. For example, one of our participants, Matthew, said this after a heart attack:

> It got to the stage that I knew I was going to die and that was the turning point. I knew I was going to die unless I did something about it. And then I just got into gear and it turned me right around.

> (Matthew)

But this was after his fourth heart attack, aged 37; the first, second and third heart attacks had not had the same impact. Other factors had to have been involved. What might these be?

Recognising that behaviour is the problem

Many people who are overweight believe in a biological cause of their weight problem, saying, 'It runs in my family', 'I have a slow metabolism', 'I was born like this', 'It's my hormones' or 'My diabetes makes me overweight'. Although there is some evidence that weight is, in part, influenced by biology and forces beyond our control, this way of thinking does not help us change our behaviour, as we believe that there is nothing we can do. For example, if you believe that your heart attack was caused by 'doing too much', you will not follow advice to 'do more exercise' but will prefer to rest and relax. Likewise, if you believe 'I am overweight because of my biology', you will not try to eat less, as this does not match. We only adopt solutions to a problem if they match our beliefs about the cause. This is illustrated by one of our participants who had never managed to lose weight and keep it off:

> I was born overweight, and I've always been overweight. . . . I was a fat child and then a fat teenager and fat adult and my weight has never decreased, it always just went up. . . I was never a normal weight.
>
> (Julie)

In contrast, people who have successfully lost weight and kept it off hold a more behavioural model of both the cause of their weight problem, 'I overeat', and the solution, 'I need to eat less'; their model is coherent and emphasises behaviour. For example, as one participant who has lost and maintained this loss described how his problem had been caused by:

> drinking too much ... eating for comfort ... lived in a house where there was always much too much to eat ... finishing off children's food.
>
> (David)

Sometimes this shift towards a behavioural model of body weight may be triggered by the life event itself, or it may come about through something the person has read or seen or as a response to an intervention by a health professional. For example, if someone recognises that they lost weight last time they were ill and gained it whilst on holiday, the link between eating and weight starts to become clearer.

Disrupting the cost-benefit analysis

Most behaviours are governed by a simple cost-benefit analysis, and eating behaviour is no different. Successful weight loss seems to occur when the benefits of the old, unhealthy habits no longer outweigh the costs, and at times, this can be the result of a life event. For example, if someone loses their job, they no longer get the benefits of eating cakes from the food trolley or having a large pub lunch with colleagues. Similarly, if their marriage breaks up, food need no longer be their way to manage a problematic relationship. One man who had lost weight described how this had happened after he had split up with his 'monster of a girlfriend':

> Before we split up, I would be happy, then we would have a row or something and I would think, 'Oh, I can't be bothered, I will go out and eat McDonald's'. But after we split up I was back home with my family, I was seeing my friends a lot more… I wanted to look good. I wanted to look good naked, that's what I used to say to myself'.

> (Jack)

The life event had taken away his need to overeat (as he was no longer arguing with his girlfriend) and changed where he lived and who he was living with.

Bringing the costs into the here and now

People are very good at future discounting and will ignore future costs in favour of focusing on any benefits in the here and now. For eating, this can be problematic as the benefits of eating are always immediate, whereas the costs are always in the months and years to come. Sometimes, life events can change the timing of these costs and benefits by making the costs seem more immediate. For example, if the life event is a health crisis such as a heart attack or a diagnosis of diabetes, then the costs of unhealthy eating are no longer way ahead in the future but have been brought into the here and now, making them harder to ignore. This is also the case with setting achievable goals, such as eating regularly or cooking meals rather than snacking. One such goal could be helped by self-weighing, as this enables the individual to gain regular rewards from sticking to their eating plan. As one of our participants said:

I go every week to get weighed. Tonight's our night and I'll go tonight to get weighed even though I'm on night shift and I know my weight will be different because I'm on night duty. I will still go and get weighed because I don't want to get out of my target range.

(Mandy)

Successful dieting is, therefore, not only about disrupting the cost-benefit analysis but also about changing the timing of these factors.

Investment in success

Weight loss can be extremely hard work as it involves changing habits that have been ingrained for a lifetime, existing in a state of denial, missing out on social events and changing the way people live their day-to-day lives. It is sometimes difficult to understand how, when people have been through all this, they put the weight back on, only to have to start the struggle all over again. But fortunately, in many ways, we are not good at remembering difficult episodes in our lives and over time, these memories fade, which is helpful for traumatic events but not helpful for dieting, as people slip back into their old habits and the weight is regained. Weight loss maintenance seems more likely to occur after initial weight loss if people recognise and can remember how difficult this initial stage was. As one woman said:

I've worked hard to get it off. . . I don't want to go back.

(Kerri)

One participant described how she used photos of herself to remember how hard losing weight had been:

I have pictures of how I used to look stuck up in the bedroom, I've got them stuck on my fridge and inside the cupboard to remind me … when I'm thinking oh, I could eat some rubbish, and I am thinking, no. You are not going to start that again.

(Emily)

This is a form of investment that, if emphasised, stored, focused on and kept salient, can help weight loss maintenance. There are many strategies that can be used to strengthen the sense of investment, such as keeping a diary, filling in a checklist of suffering or writing a list of suffering and placing it in a public place.

A new identity and the process of reinvention

Successful dieters seem to develop a new identity around being a thinner, healthier person, making it harder for them to regain their lost weight, as this would no longer be in line with how they see themselves. For some, this new sense of self can be incorporated into their existing life, but for many it involves a process of reinvention and the establishment of a new way of being, which manifests itself in becoming something like a gym instructor, a personal trainer, a nutritionist or an organiser for a weight loss group or in taking up triathlons or marathons. Our participants have called this many things, including 'a new start', 'a rebirth', 'a new me' and 'a last chance'. As one man said:

> I feel more confident... I'm less embarrassed and not self-conscious anymore and body language has changed... I can just lean back in my chair and talk... I feel like I've got a new life, new chances, new opportunities. I'm a new person... It is rebirth really. (Michael)

And once this new identity has been created, it makes it much more likely that any weight loss will be maintained.

No more emotional eating

Being overweight can often be the result of emotional eating, and food is used to regulate our emotions. As one of our participants said of food:

> I use it so much to control my emotions although of course it never does and makes it worse. It's not a friend but it's an emotional support... I have a sort of love/hate relationship with food. (Sophie)

Successful dieters often talk about finding alternative coping mechanisms, which can include exercise, talking to friends, singing, playing a musical instrument or finding a new hobby. As one woman said:

> I go and sit in the bath, and I'm learning to deal with my emotions differently. (Julie)

And another said:

> You still do think about it [food], because you don't want to go back where you were, and so you think, what you need to do is occupy your mind, go out for a walk, because when you're out for a walk you can't open the fridge door, so it's a case of occupying your mind. (Peter)

Finding a substitute coping mechanism is not easy, though, and several participants have described their struggle to find alternative behaviours:

> If you've used food as your comfort, your security blanket, as your friend, then how do you deal with it if you can't use that anymore? There's no mechanism for me as to how I should deal with things apart from eating. (Saara)

And for some, their chosen substitute behaviour can also be unhealthy. As one of our patients after bariatric surgery said:

> Post surgery, I definitely transferred to alcohol 'cos I couldn't eat... It was easier and easier to drink to fulfil the need in me. (Jade)

A new eating routine

Part of losing weight for the long term is the establishment of a new, healthier routine which can persist forever onwards, rather than just in the short term. As one successful dieter described:

> You've got to change your — the way you're eating for a life; it's not just, you know, for a period of time, it's permanent. You've got to make a permanent change, and it's what I've done. (Jane)

Different success stories involve a wide range of new and different eating habits, and there is no one-size-fits-all eating habit that fits all. However, when weight loss is maintained this is most often associated with eating a healthier diet, which is higher in fruit and vegetables and lower in calories. As one woman said:

> I eat more salads, more vegetables, more pickles … I eat plates of boiled vegetables and I eat a lot of salads. I like that. I put horseradish with it sometimes. Sometimes chilli sauce … everything I eat now is either brown or natural. (Sarah)

One woman also described how her own healthier eating habits had also influenced the rest of her family:

> We don't go to McDonald's anymore, we don't have pizzas. We used to go to Greggs and buy donuts and we don't do that… Me and my family are being healthy now. (Angela)

Successful dieting seems to be linked to new habits which can be sustained in the longer term, which also involves changing the habits of others.

Feeling in control

Many people who have lost weight and kept it off describe a new sense of control over food. For those who have used more traditional dieting approaches, this comes from the development of new habits, a reduction in emotional eating due to new alternative coping strategies and a shift in their beliefs about food and the role it plays in their lives. It is also reflected in feeling able to have a level of flexible control rather than seeing food as forbidden or banned:

> We have our little treats, I have had biscuits … I don't feel deprived of anything. If I want a chocolate I can have it. You just count it. I can actually still eat quite a lot of the meals I used to eat and I have enjoyed a cooked breakfast this week. The fact that I can eat all this, it's tasty and I feel like I am enjoying normal food, not diet food. (Emily)

Some people lose weight through surgery. This can often be accompanied by a change in control. For those people, a regained sense of control was paradoxically a result of feeling that their choices over food had been taken out of their hands as the operation was limiting their food intake for them. I have called this the 'paradox of control' as by taking away control, surgery can make people feel more in control:

> Now I feel that the control is taken out of my hands. I didn't have that control over my body because my stomach controlled everything. If I eat too much, I'm sick so I don't have the control anymore … that's a good thing because I couldn't control on my own. (Jenny)

People do not have to have surgery to feel like this. Simply not bringing food into the home can help.

Finding hope that the future can be different

The final factor that seems to relate to successful weight loss and maintenance is hope. Most people carry on their day-to-day lives in a habitual way and see their future lives as being very much like the past and present. This is fine for those who are healthy and happy and can lead to contentment and well-being. But for those who are not, it leads to getting stuck. One way to become unstuck is to find a sense of hope that there is another possible future out there, which is different and better than the one that has been mapped out for years. For dieters, this sense of hope can come from hearing other people's success stories, taking full credit for times in their own lives when they have changed their behaviour or monitoring their behaviour to find small signs of change to offer hope that change is possible. One of our patients described to us the moment she realised there was hope that her future could be better than her past, and it involved seeing an image of her body during a scan at a hospital:

> My orthopaedic surgeon got a bone scan … he's like my body there and there's me, there's all my fat, and he goes to the kids, 'Look, there's a little Mummy in there trying to get out'. You know, there is a little me here … seeing it on the bone scan … that's when I decided to go for it. (Julie)

For this woman, the image of the 'little me' version of herself gave her hope, which in turn resulted in her changing her behaviour and losing weight.

In-depth accounts of success stories are one approach to discovering the mechanisms behind successful dieting and indicate a number of processes. These accounts illustrate that longer-term changes in behaviour can be sustained and that these can lead to weight loss. These stories also shed light on which factors make this success more likely to come about.

In summary

Research has explored the different ways in which people manage to change their behaviour, lose weight and sometimes manage to keep it off. This has focused on quantitative research and people's own stories and highlights a role for factors such as an initial trigger, the belief that things can change, a shift in the cost-benefit analysis for eating and exercise, a new behaviour regimen, a sense of hope and control and a new identity all of which together make the person less likely to revert back to their old behaviours.

HOW CAN I CHANGE MY BEHAVIOUR AND LOSE WEIGHT IN THE LONG TERM?

Given the findings from this research, what does this mean if you want to change your diet to lose weight? Using the approaches described above, there are clearly overlapping factors that keep reappearing and are linked to successful behaviour change and weight loss. Beyond variables such as being male, being older and having a higher initial body weight, which seem to relate to success but are fixed, all this evidence illustrates that there are seven key factors which can be used to explain how some people manage to lose weight and keep it off. These factors are all relevant to those who are trying to lose weight whether it be through changing their behaviour, having weight loss surgery or taking weight loss medication.

Triggered by a life event: First, successful changes in behaviour are often **triggered by a life event,** which shakes up the person's world and offers a chance for change. This may be a diagnosis, such as a heart attack or diabetes, an injury, such as knee pain or a back problem, a change of life status, such as a divorce or separation or a house move or even just the recognition that something has changed, such as struggling to put on shoes or get out of the bath. These events shake up the person's status quo and offer up the chance to change. Sometimes people respond to these events by trying to keep things as they are and re-establish their equilibrium, but for others, this is the nudge they need to start to reinvent themselves. This offers up a new space for the person to bring about change. It also often creates a change in some of the factors that were encouraging less healthy behaviours in the first place, such as negative social support. This can often change what is in our heads in terms of our beliefs about ourselves, our body weight and our behaviour. They can also change our environment in terms of the people around us and the world we encounter in our daily lives.

Believing things can change and having hope: Second, if the person also believes in a behavioural model of their weight problem and has **hope that things can change,** this makes an initial change more likely. For example, whilst many people believe in a biological model of body weight and feel that there is nothing they can do, this medical model can become a self-fulfilling prophecy – people think there is nothing they can do, so they do not feel able to do anything. In contrast, however, if people can be encouraged to take a more psychological model of their weight, then they can feel empowered to bring about a change. There is a downside to a psychological model in that it can be associated with stigma and blame – believing body weight can change but not actually changing it can lead others to be judgmental, and the person themselves can feel a failure. But with some reframing and support, a more psychological model can lead to a sense of agency and power. So rather than being a victim of their uncontrollable biology or an environment that is working against them, people can start to feel some hope that there is something they can do for themselves, rather than being a victim of their biology. To shift towards a sense of hope that things can change, ask yourself these questions about your body weight. Ask: 'Have I ever lost weight?' If the answer is, 'yes, when I was poorly last year with flu', consider whether this was because you went off your food and ate less. Also ask, 'Have I ever just put on a lot of weight?' If the answer is 'yes, in Greece on holiday', consider whether this was because you went out for dinner more and ate all the lovely Greek food. Hopefully, these questions start to show that body weight cannot just be biology and must be linked to what you do! This is empowering.

A shift in the cost-benefit analysis: The third factor that can facilitate successful weight loss is a **shift in the cost-benefit analysis** of health behaviours. Most behaviours at their simplest are just the result of a simple cost-benefit analysis – exercise is fun but tiring; going to the gym is sociable but costs money; eating well requires planning and time but makes me feel better about myself; eating out is sociable but often involves lots of calories. Added to this is the tendency to show future discounting, so benefits in the here and now will often outweigh costs in the future – so thinking 'I like eating takeaways now' will often beat the risk of a heart attack in the future. This shift in the cost-benefit analysis can be brought about by focusing on the more immediate consequences of weight loss, such as improved body image, being able to wear different clothes, getting positive feedback from others, feeling less breathless or having less joint pain. It can come about by disrupting some of the costs to behaviour change, such as a change in job or relationship, if people have been delivering negative social support, such as sabotage, collusion or moving house away from the chip shop. It can also come about by finding new benefits to behaviour change, such as eating alone after a divorce from a difficult partner or finding new friends to do exercise with, in a new job. This shift in balance can also be brought about through strategies, such as goal setting and making specific plans to shop or cook differently or be more active or contact a formal intervention or dietician to gain regular feedback and support. Such changes not only enable healthier behaviours to have greater benefits but also bring these benefits into the here and now, making them more sustainable.

An initial investment: Fourth, successful behavioural change and sustained weight loss also seem to need the person to have made an initial **investment** in change. The mantra 'try, try, try again and at last, you will succeed' seems to be true for weight loss. This is illustrated by the role of dieting attempts in the past being predictive of success in the future. This investment also seems to help give momentum to their ongoing success. Therefore, if someone loses a lot of weight at first, which involves a lot of effort and determination, then they are more likely to feel 'I have tried so hard and put so much into this process, I might as well continue'. We carried out a series of studies encouraging people to focus on the investment they had already made in terms of their time, money, effort, relationships, sacrifices, etc., and there was some evidence that this could help people sustain and any changes they had made as they became more aware of the effort it had taken to get so far (14,15).

A new behaviour regimen: We are creatures of habit, and for any changes in weight that are to be maintained, new habits need to be formed, which can carry on into the future. For those who are able to lose weight and keep it off, this is sustained by a **new consistent behaviour regimen** which often consists of breakfast, regular mealtimes, healthy eating and a reduced intake of fat, together with increased physical activity. These behaviours need to be associated with certain times of day (breakfast, lunch and dinner) to help avoid snacking and emotional eating and can be helped with regular planning so that people know what they are going to eat and when. These behaviours also need to be associated with certain places, such as the kitchen table, local café, the common room or the dining room, to encourage mindful eating and to avoid eating on the go and should be thought of as 'meals', not 'snacks', to make sure they are as filling as possible.

A renewed sense of control: This process is also supported by a **renewed sense of control,** sometimes helped through self-monitoring such as keeping a diary or having a sticker chart, which in turn, leads to healthier behaviours. This process also feeds itself, as when someone starts to change their behaviours and lose weight, they feel better about themselves, which in turn boosts their confidence and sense of empowerment and control, which makes continued change easier to manage.

A new identity: After losing weight, many people can still feel that they are still a fatter person in a thinner person's body, which can make them doubt themselves and feel uncomfortable with who they have become. This can also be exacerbated by negative social support if friends, family members or partners do not want them to change and criticise their new shape rather than celebrating with them. This can lead to a sense of imposter syndrome, guilt or lowered self-esteem, which in turn can lead to overeating and slipping backwards to where other people would prefer them to be. Others, however, who manage to show successful dieting seem to develop a **new identity** through a process of reinvention, at the centre of which is a healthier, thinner self. For some, this can involve becoming the leader of their local weight loss group, a personal trainer or a spokesperson for weight management. This involves a level of commitment to their new self, which makes it harder to lapse back to who they were. Others manage to embrace their new self without this level of public commitment but draw upon other sources of support, such as new jobs, new relationships, new clothes or new hobbies that enable them to embrace this new version of themselves.

Avoiding rebound effects: We know from research on food parenting that buying unhealthy food but not letting a child eat it (overt control) can make the child more preoccupied with that food and simply want it more. We also know from dieting research that trying not to eat foods that you still want to eat can create the 'what the hell effect' and ultimately trigger overeating (16, 17). Together, these are both examples of rebound effects when trying not to do something ultimately makes you do it more. This is extremely problematic for any attempt to change eating behaviour, and mostly, this happens because we put ourselves into a state of denial, which can only last for a short time and ultimately results in eating more. Avoiding rebound effects is therefore central to successful behaviour change. All of the factors described above can help to avoid rebound effects as they reduce the need for denial, take away some of the benefits of eating more, add to the benefits of eating less and help to create investment in a future self, embedded with a healthier identity, which makes it harder to relapse back to how things used to be.

In summary

Successful dieting has been explored using quantitative research and listening to people's stories. Across these different approaches are several common factors which seem to facilitate sustained weight loss. These involve an initial trigger, the belief that things can change, a shift in the cost-benefit analysis for eating and exercise, a new behaviour regimen, a sense of control and a new identity, all of which together make the person less likely to revert to their old behaviours. This offers lessons learned that can also be applied to making daily changes to diet to be healthier, rather than for weight loss.

HOW CAN I CHANGE MY DIET TO BE HEALTHIER (WITHOUT MAKING FOOD INTO A PROBLEM)?

Whilst wanting to lose weight is a very common motivation behind dietary change, many people also want to eat well through eating more fruit and vegetables, snacking less, eating fewer ultra-processed foods or cutting out meat. Changing behaviour in these ways is open to many of the common pitfalls of dieting including an increased preoccupation with the very foods trying to be avoided, falling back into old habits, short term changes in behaviour that do not last and compensatory behaviours whereby people might be healthier in one area of their lives but become less healthy in others (e.g. eating more vegetables but also eating more meat; snacking less but doing less exercise; stopping eating meat but eating ultra processed meat substitutes or just chocolate). What lessons can we learn from the evidence about how to make these other changes to your diet in ways that last, do not cause rebound effects and can help you to have a good relationship with food?

Choosing the right moment to change

Successful dieting often happens after a life event such as a heart attack or divorce. Other changes in your diet are also easier to make if you choose the right time to start, and this can often be after something else has changed in your life. For example, if you have started a new relationship, this could be a time to eat more fruit and vegetables, cut down on meat and snack less. Likewise, if you have changed jobs, then you could stop eating at your desk, start taking in a healthier lunch box or buy healthier food from the local noodle bar. Or if you have moved flat or had a new kitchen built, then use this opportunity to find a new place to eat, enjoy a different place to cook and fill your fridge with different types of food. This will give your decision to make a change a sense of renewal, excitement and investment that can help it get underway.

Believing things can change

In a similar way that many people think their body weight is fixed by their biology, people also feel that some foods simply 'taste better' and that food preferences are fixed by their taste buds. They might also believe that they must snack in between meals, or they will be starving, or that they feel too bloated after eating vegetables. Whilst different people do have different reactions to foods, and some have intolerances or even allergies, many of our beliefs about food simply come from what we are used to and the habits we have built up over our lifetime. To change our behaviour, we therefore need to believe that it can be changed. One way to do this is to ask ourselves questions to challenge our beliefs. Ask, 'Do I eat the same food and at the same times as I did 10 years ago?'. If the answer is 'No' because you eat out more (more money?), cook more (I was bought a cookery book for my birthday and found I enjoyed it), snack more (my job is really busy) or eat more kids' foods (I have kids now and finish their leftovers) then you can see that your diet can change. And if it has changed, it can change again. This should give you greater hope for a healthier future.

A shift in the cost-benefit analysis

If you want to snack less, eat less meat, eat more fruit and vegetables or cook more, then these changes can be achieved by shifting the costs and benefits of these behaviours. First, I would suggest making small, manageable changes, not huge ones. So, if you do not eat many vegetables, try carrots, parsnips or red peppers, rather than artichokes or fennel, which are more of an acquired taste. Then try frozen bags or preprepared vegetables that are easy to cook, rather than time-consuming gourmet varieties, which can take more effort than they are worth. Likewise, if you want to cook more, keep it simple and fun, lower your expectations and do not watch too many cookery programmes. Pretty much anything home-cooked from scratch (even if it is pasta pesto and salad) is better than a ready meal or takeaway (see the recipes at the end of this book). Keeping it simple reduces the costs of trying something new and increases the chance of there being a benefit. Second, focus on the immediate benefits in the here and now. Eating more vegetables is good for your health and protects you from all sorts of health conditions. But do not expect to see any of these health benefits in the short term. BUT you will see other more immediate benefits, such as clearer skin, better sleep, stronger nails and a more regular and satisfying digestive system! Likewise, you will also save money now if you cook simply from scratch and do not eat out or buy takeaways. Then, what is good about building a new habit is that after a while, you will start to feel an immediate cost if you do not eat vegetables with each meal, if you do not cook or if you do buy an ultra-processed ready meal which will suddenly taste plastic and full of chemicals! Small changes can shift the cost-benefit analysis, and by focusing on the benefits in the here and now, after a while, your old, unhealthier behaviour will start to feel as if something is missing.

Remind yourself of the investment you have made

One of the tricks about sustaining any new habit is to focus on the effort you have put in so far. So, if you have been cooking more, eating more vegetables or eating less meat, put a chart on the fridge to keep a record of what you have tried, tell others how good you have become, treat yourself at the end of each week to celebrate your successes and generally revel in how well you have done. Even keep a score of how much money you have not spent on takeaways and think of better ways to spend it. This level of investment, then conscientiously focusing on the level of investment, makes it much harder to slip back into old ways.

Create a new behaviour regimen

We are all creatures of habit, which are a product of repetition, reinforcement and association. Old habits are, therefore, difficult to break because they have become almost automatic and we do them often without much thought. Changing our diets to eat more healthily involves learning new habits, which is helped through all the processes described so far – choosing the right time, believing things can change, shifting the cost-benefit analysis and focusing on the investment made so far. Then, once these processes have started to happen, the new changes need to be embedded into our lives to become the new habits and replace the old ones. At its most basic, this involves repetition (just keep doing it again and again), reinforcement (praise yourself, keep a sticker chart, get praise from others, focus on the immediate benefits) and association (pairing the new foods with thoughts of a healthy digestion, imagining improvements to your heart, even looking at your healthier poo!). But this process of establishing new habits can also be helped by strategies such as planning (having a shopping list, meal planning), setting yourself reasonable goals (five home cooked meals a week, at least frozen mixed veg with every dinner), finding good role models to copy (your parents, a friend, a chef who cooks feasible not elaborate meals, a celebrity you like) and managing your environment (buy in the food you want to eat, don't buy the food you don't want to eat, don't go to unhealthy cafes, don't go down the unhealthy food isles). Then just keep going. And soon, like all habits, this will become your new normal, and you will miss it and feel strange if you slip back to your old ways.

Create a new sense of self

One of the best ways to keep a new habit going is to become invested in the idea that this is who you now are – your new sense of self. For some, this can mean becoming a health influencer who is passionate about vegetarianism, someone who writes an online blog about eating vegetables or a health guru who sells cookery books. They become so wedded to their new identity that they can never go back to who they were before – the loss would be too great. But for most of us, our lives pretty much carry on as they did before; we just eat differently! But it is still useful to celebrate this new sense of self by telling others how well you have done, inviting people round for dinner so they can see how you now cook from scratch and encouraging those close to you to tell others that you have managed to eat three different types of vegetables in the past week. We all need praise and recognition, and the more we become proud of our new habits and the more they become a part of how we see ourselves, the more likely they are to stick.

And all this to avoid rebound effects

When people try to eat less, they can end up eating more as they crave the foods they are trying to avoid (16,17). The same can happen when trying to eat more healthily – takeaways, fast food, processed meals and meat can all seem more desirable once we try not to eat them. All of the processes described above can help prevent a rebound effect so when we chose the best time to make a change, believe that change is possible, create a shift in the costs-benefit analysis, focus on the investment made, manage to create a new behaviour regimen and develop a sense of identity which focuses on a healthier self than rebound is much less likely to happen. But in addition, it helps if we just do not want to eat that way anymore. From my experience, whilst dieters may crave cake, vegetarians rarely crave meat as they see it as disgusting or immoral, and most adults rarely crave the brightly coloured sweets from their childhoods, as they are seen as bad for their teeth. So, to help with building a new eating habit, first focus on the new foods to eat in a positive way to avoid denial – 'I will eat more fruit and vegetables', 'I will eat more home-cooked foods' and 'I will eat a more varied diet' rather than thinking about what you will not eat. Then, if you can, reframe the foods you are trying to avoid as undesirable (rather than desirable but to be avoided) – they are unhealthy, full of chemicals, full of sugar and salt, bad for my digestion, and bad for my skin. Then, finally, try not to demonise anything. All foods are OK in moderation, and if you do find you have slipped back into old ways, do not be too critical of yourself. Just start again with your new ways on the day after.

In summary

Whilst some people want to change their diet to lose weight, many just want to improve their diet and eat more healthily. This can be achieved using the lessons learned from successful dieting and applying them to other changes, such as eating more fruit and vegetables, cooking more or eating less meat. In essence, this means choosing the right time to change, believing that things can change, shifting the cost-benefit analysis, focusing on the investment made so far, creating a new behaviour regimen and embedding all these changes into a new sense of self that becomes part of who you are. Together, these processes help to avoid any rebound effects and make new habits more likely to be sustained in the long term.

To conclude

This chapter has explored how people can change what they eat, first by focusing on the research evidence for longer-term behaviour change and weight loss; then examining how this evidence can be applied to making and sustaining changes in behaviour to lose weight. Then, finally, the chapter outlined the key lessons learned from the evidence to make daily changes to be healthier in other ways, such as eating more fruit and vegetables, snacking less, eating less meat or consuming fewer ultra-processed foods. In essence, changing eating habits for whatever reason is about building a new eating regimen whilst avoiding rebound effects. Factors that help this include choosing the right time to start a change, believing that things can change, shifting the cost-benefit analysis to focus on immediate benefits, and creating a new identity based on this healthier self. That way, eating behaviours can be changed for the long term without making food into a problem.

REFERENCES

1. Wing, R.R., and Phelan, S. (2005). Long-term weight loss maintenance. *American Journal of Clinical Nutrition*, 82(Supplement 1), 222S–225S. Review. PubMed PMID: 16002825.
2. Ogden, J. (2000). The correlates of long terms weight loss: A group comparison study of obesity. *International Journal of Obesity*, 24, 1018–1025.
3. Elfhag, K., and Rössner, S. (2005). Who succeeds in maintaining weight loss? A conceptual review of factors associated with weight loss maintenance and weight regain. *Obesity Reviews*, 6(1), 67–85.
4. Epiphaniou, E., and Ogden, J. (2010). Evaluating the role of triggers and sustaining conditions in weight loss maintenance. *Journal of Obesity*, 8594143 Open Access. doi: 10.1155/2010/859413.

5. Thomas, J.G., Bond, D.S., Phelan, S., Hill, J.O., and Wing, R.R. (2014). Weight-loss maintenance for 10 years in the National Weight Control Registry. *American Journal of Preventive Medicine*, 46(1), 17–23.

6. Stubbs, J., Whybrow, S., Teixeira, P., Blundell, J., Lawton, C., Westenhoefer, J., ...Raats, M. (2011). Problems in identifying predictors and correlates of weight loss and maintenance: Implications for weight control therapies based on behaviour change. *Obesity Reviews*, 12(9), 688–708.

7. Hartmann-Boyce, J., Johns, D.J., Jebb, S.A., and Aveyard, P. (2014). Behavioural weight management review group: Effect of behavioural techniques and delivery mode on effectiveness of weight management: Systematic review, meta-analysis and meta-regression. *Obesity Reviews*, 15(7), 598–609.

8. Ogden, J., and Sidhu, S. (2006). Adherence, behaviour change and visualisation: A qualitative study of patient's experiences of obesity medication. *The Journal of Psychosomatic Research*, 61, 545–552.

9. Ogden, J., and Hills, L. (2008). Understanding sustained changes in behaviour: The role of life events and the process of reinvention. *Health: An International Journal*, 12, 419–437.

10. Epiphaniou, E., and Ogden, J. (2010). Successful weight loss maintenance: From a restricted to liberated self. *International Journal of Health Psychology*, 15, 887–896.

11. Ogden, J., Clementi, C., and Aylwin, S. (2006). Having obesity surgery: A qualitative study and the paradox of control. *Psychology and Health*, 21, 273–293.

12. Wood, K., and Ogden, J. (2016). Obesity Patients' long-term experiences following obesity surgery with a focus on eating behaviour: A qualitative study. *Journal of Health Psychology*, 21(11), 2447–2456.

13. Greaves, C., Poltawski, L., Garside, R., and Briscoe, S. (2017). Understanding the challenge of weight loss maintenance: A systematic review and synthesis of qualitative research on weight loss maintenance. *Health Psychology Review*, 11(2), 1–19. doi: 10.1080/17437199.2017.1299583

14. Husted, M., and Ogden, J. (2014). Impact of an investment based intervention on weight-loss and hedonic thoughts about food post-obesity surgery. *Journal of Obesity*, 810374. doi:10.1155/2014/810374

15. Hollywood, A., Ogden, J., and Hashemi, M. (2023). A randomised control trial assessing the impact of an investment-based intervention on weight-loss, glycated haemoglobin and psychological outcomes 1 year post

bariatric surgery. *NIHR Open Research*, 3:27, https://doi.org/10.3310/nihr openres.13408.1

16. Polivy, J., and Herman, C.P. (1999). Distress and eating: Why do dieters overeat? *International Journal of Eating Disorders*, 26, 153–164.

17. Polivy, J., and Heatherton, T. (2015). Spiral model of dieting and disordered eating: Encyclopaedia of feeding and eating disorders. New York: Springer.

8

HOW DO I EAT WELL
AS AN ADULT?

Eating well as an adult involves developing a good relationship with food. It also helps to have a good relationship with your body size and shape. Developing a good relationship with food will be described in terms of putting food back into its box through managing the when, where, why and how of eating, avoiding emotional and mindless eating and avoiding rebound effects. Developing a good relationship with your body size is described in terms of understanding the causes of body dissatisfaction, learning to be critical of the media, managing your comparison groups and developing positive self-talk. Good strategies that can help towards both these goals involve planning (mostly better than spur of the moment decisions), self-monitoring (keeping a diary), finding substitutes (dancing, not eating), rescripting (finding the positive reframe) and taking perspective (what would someone else say). It also helps to aim high but be kind to yourself if things do not quite work out.

HOW CAN I HAVE A GOOD RELATIONSHIP
WITH FOOD?

Chapter 1 described what it means to eat well at every age and explored what, when, where, why and how we can eat in a way that

DOI: 10.4324/9781003600183-13

is good for both our physical and mental health. Having a good relationship with food as an adult involves managing the what, when, where, why and how of eating. It also involves putting food back into its box, avoiding emotional and mindless eating, avoiding rebound effects and being kind to yourself.

Managing the what, when, where, why and how of eating

For the what: healthy eating in essence is about eating a varied diet which is high in fruit and vegetables, moderate in protein and complex carbohydrates such as brown bread, pasta and rice and low in sugary and ultra-processed foods. A useful shorthand for eating a varied diet is to 'eat the rainbow', a tool to avoid ultra-processed foods is to cook from scratch whenever possible, and a trick to generally improve your diet is to snack less (as snacks tend to be sugary/salty/ultra-processed). It is also useful to keep food simple, watch fewer TV chefs, have 'good enough' standards and avoid ready meals and takeaways. Cooking for 20 minutes is pretty much always better than reheating a ready meal for 15. There are some easy and quick recipes at the end of this book.

For the when and where: eating at designated times and places throughout the day helps to promote eating well in many ways. First, it encourages planning and thinking ahead, which means that food is considered rather than just spontaneous. Considered choices are pretty much always better than those made in the heat of the moment. Next, it encourages delayed gratification and holding any feelings of hunger rather than just eating as and when the need arises. Holding hunger enables us to enjoy eating more when it happens and to learn to tolerate hunger rather than fear it. Further, eating at a table and sitting down rather than 'on the go' makes us process the food we are eating, which can help to fill us up and remember we have eaten later in the day. And finally, eating at a time designated as 'dinner' at a place called 'the dinner table' puts food back into its box and prevents it from spilling out into every nook and cranny of our lives.

For the why of eating: many of us eat for reasons other than hunger. First, our childhood has often filled us up with associations between food and boredom, upset, frustration, reward, treat and distraction. Then, when adults, these associations between food and all sorts of emotions mean that we use food for emotional regulation. Emotional eating may work in the short term and can lead to a temporary relief from our low mood or even lift our mood when we want to be distracted from whatever is happening in our lives. But these benefits are often short-lived and can result in a backlash and ultimate feelings of guilt or shame. Then, for some, this can lead to further eating, and so the spiral continues. It is better, therefore, to try to recognise when we are eating for emotional reasons and find other non-food ways to manage our emotions. Second, we also just eat because it is there. The modern world provides us with food at every opportunity, whether it be at the petrol station, in the cinema, at a work meeting or on the train. This can lead to mindless eating when we eat without hunger and without any real awareness of what food we are putting into our bodies. We need to be aware of all these food cues around us and work towards eating more mindfully.

In terms of how to eat, we need to eat with awareness, with planning and at a designated space and time so that we can eat more mindfully and process what food we are putting into our bodies.

Together, managing the what, when, where, why and how of eating leads to eating well, which results not only in a healthier diet but also a far better relationship with food. All of the above helps to put food back into its box.

Putting food back into its box

Food means many things other than hunger. It means emotional regulation and is used to manage upset, boredom, anxiety, depression and loneliness. It also means social interaction and is key to how we interact at family get-togethers, religious gatherings, date nights and nights out (or in) with our friends. And it is also key to our sense of self and how we communicate this to the outside world – do we see ourselves as someone who loves food, is picky about food, eats a lot, loves cooking or cannot really be bothered? Food is also ever-present and forms part of how we travel (eating in the car, the train, the plane), how we work (at our desk, in a meeting), how we relax (on the sofa, in bed) and how we entertain ourselves (at the cinema, watching sport). It has, therefore, spilt out of its box, and whilst some of this is all just part of modern living, having a good relationship with food is in part about putting it back in its box and eating as just one part of life.

Avoiding emotional and mindless eating

The key to having a good relationship with food is about avoiding both emotional and mindless eating. So how can this be achieved?

The main way to manage both emotional and mindless eating is to work out when you are eating and why, which can be simply achieved through keeping a diary. So, sort out either an online or paper diary and each day write down what you eat, where you eat and then what the triggers were and how you were feeling. As the days and weeks pass, you can then start to look for patterns to see what emotional or environmental factors are related to what you eat.

Once these factors have been identified, you then need to find substitutes and alternative ways to manage these triggers. For example, if you find that you are eating when you are bored to just distract yourself or do something with your hands, find some other form of distraction such as a fidget board, texting a friend or going for a quick walk. If you are eating when you are upset, try an alternative to lift your mood, such as listening to music, having a dance around the kitchen, calling a friend for a chat or having a bath. If you are eating because food is just there, then try not to buy food and bring it into the house if you do not want to eat it. Buy ingredients that need cooking, not snacks, and plan what and when you are going to eat so you do not eat in between meals. Or if you are buying food from the shops that you do not want to eat, take a shopping list with you, avoid the 'unhealthy' shopping aisles, shop when you are not hungry, shop online and make life easier for yourself by making it harder to eat just because it is there.

Then, when you do eat, eat at a table, sitting down, off a plate with a knife and fork and think mindfully, 'I am having a meal' and then think about what you are eating rather than being distracted by the TV or your phone.

Food will never be just about hunger and our biological need for nutrients, but it can be about less than it is for most people at the moment. And making it less about emotional eating and learning to eat more mindfully is a step towards developing a good relationship with food.

Avoiding rebound effects

We live in a world where many foods have been demonised and food is often seen as 'good vs bad', 'healthy vs unhealthy' or 'fattening vs slimming'. This dichotomous view can result in certain foods being avoided and sometimes even cut out of the diet. For example, there have been fads for 'low-fat diets' when people grilled everything; for low-carbohydrate diets when fried eggs were in vogue and for high-protein diets when everyone seemed to eat meat. When food is classified in this way, it can lead to periods of denial, which can ultimately lead to craving, rebound effects and overeating. Rebound effects are not only unhealthy in terms of what and why we eat, but can also lead to feelings of failure, guilt and shame, which are not good for wellbeing. Eating well as an adult is therefore best achieved through a moderation approach to most foods and by rescripting foods from 'good vs bad' to 'better vs worse' or 'frequent vs occasional'. And this often requires the ability to be kind to yourself.

Being kind to yourself

Aim high, try to eat well and avoid emotional and mindless eating and rebound effects. But also accept that the world is complex, you are an emotional being, and the food industry is not always our friend. Then, when things do not go your way, be kind to yourself. Eating well is about trying to eat well, but accepting that it is not realistic or even desirable to do this all the time. You can have meals out, the odd snack, meals in front of the TV and even the odd ready meal. Self-compassion is the cornerstone of any well-being intervention and has been linked to many positive physical and mental health outcomes (1). It is also key to changing behaviour and self-care and avoiding rebound effects. So, when you have made a plan but not followed it, or have not even made a plan, accept that this has happened, understand why it has happened, forgive yourself and carry on.

In summary

Eating well is about so much more than what food we put into our bodies and involves developing a good relationship with food, where food is a part of life but not everything. This means putting food back into its box and aiming high, but being kind to yourself if things do not quite work out.

HOW CAN I HAVE A GOOD RELATIONSHIP WITH MY BODY SIZE AND SHAPE?

Many people are critical of the way they look, particularly their body size and shape. This can lead to body dissatisfaction, which can result in lowered mood and self-esteem and unhealthy changes in eating behaviour. It can also sometimes lead to problematic eating (see Chapter 1). Building a good relationship with your body involves understanding the causes of body dissatisfaction, learning to be critical of the media, managing your comparison groups, developing positive self-talk and being kind to yourself.

What is body dissatisfaction?

Body dissatisfaction can be conceptualised in three different ways (2). First, it can be seen as a discrepancy between individuals' perception of their body size and their real body size, which can be detected using distorting mirrors or cameras to assess how large someone's body really is compared to how large they think it is. Second, it is sometimes measured as the discrepancy between how someone perceives their body size compared to their ideal body size, which can be assessed using body silhouettes and asking people to rate where they see themselves vs what they would like to be. Third, it may simply be negative feelings about aspects of the body, such as its size and shape. This can be assessed by questions to see whether people feel that their thighs are too wobbly or breasts are too small, and can be assessed using questions, such as, 'Do you worry about parts of your body being too big?' or 'How satisfied are you with your shoulders/breasts/chest/face/nose/stomach, etc'.

In general, women are more dissatisfied with their bodies than men, and would prefer their chests to be larger and their legs, stomachs, hips, thighs, bottoms and overall body shape to be smaller. But men also show body dissatisfaction. Research indicates that men are primarily worried about their penis size, body weight, height and muscularity. Further, studies suggest that in general, men would prefer their arms, chests and shoulders to be larger and their stomachs and overall body to be smaller. Although those with an eating disorder or weight problem show body dissatisfaction, it has become increasingly clear that body dissatisfaction is common amongst people of all shapes and sizes (2,3).

What causes body dissatisfaction?

The media: The most commonly held belief in both the lay and academic communities is that body dissatisfaction is a response to representations of 'ideal bodies' in the media. Social media, magazines, newspapers, television, films and even novels predominantly use images of thin women to sell to women and images of muscular men to sell to men. At times, these models may be advertising body size-related items such as food and clothes, but often they promote neutral items, such as vacuum cleaners and wallpaper. Some research has directly explored the association between the media and body dissatisfaction. For example, studies show that young girls who spend more time reading popular magazines and watching television show higher levels of body dissatisfaction (4). Studies have also shown that asking men and women to examine images of thin men and women from the media for just a few minutes in the laboratory can make them feel more dissatisfied with the way they look (5,6). Imagine what long-term exposure over many years could do. Research indicates that the media influences body dissatisfaction through two key processes: social comparison and internalisation (7,8). In particular, people compare themselves to these unrealistic images, which creates a discrepancy between how they see themselves and how they want to look, which in turn generates self-criticism. They then internalise these images as the norm, which means this process of upward comparison continues into their day-to-day lives.

The home environment: Research has also explored the impact of the home environment on body dissatisfaction and indicates a key role for the mother's own body dissatisfaction on that of her daughter, as well as the mother-daughter relationship. Studies indicate that there is a strong concordance between mothers who have higher body criticism and their daughters' own levels of body dissatisfaction. Some, although less research, also highlights a link with fathers' body image and that of their daughters and sons (9-11).

There are several possible mechanisms for this. At its simplest, children may just model their own behaviour and beliefs on those of their parents. Therefore, watching their mother trying to lose weight, change their body shape or weight themselves may create a negative role model that then translates into the daughter's own behaviour (9-11). Second, this process of transmission from parent to child may take place via language and the words used within a family. This approach has been explored with a focus on 'scripts', 'fat talk' or 'body talk' and the ways in which words are used and then internalised within families. For example, one study explored the used of body scripts within parent and daughter dyads and explored the use of words such as 'beautiful', 'healthy', 'slim', 'pretty', 'good looking' vs more negative ones such as 'fat', 'underweight', 'overweight', 'too skinny', 'chubby' (9). The results showed some degree of concordance between the daughters' internal scripts and those used by their parents, indicating a transmission of scripts across generations. The results also, however, suggest that this transmission was not always automatic and often the better predictor was what the daughter remembered from their childhood rather than what the parents said they had said. This suggests that it might not only be what a parent says that is important, but also how this is processed and embedded by their child.

Third, the next mechanism underpinning the development of body dissatisfaction may be reinforcement, as any behaviour that receives attention, even negative attention, can be reinforced, making it more likely to happen again. In terms of body dissatisfaction, reinforcement can take the form of both words and actions, which can both create and exacerbate any sense of self-criticism. Therefore, a girl who is praised for being pretty, losing weight, fitting into a smaller size or looking like someone from the media or a boy who is praised for developing muscles, looking strong, growing tall or having a good jaw line will realise that these are regarded as important dimensions of who they are and strive harder to achieve and maintain them. Likewise, any negative reinforcers in the form of verbal criticisms (you look fat, that doesn't fit properly, why can't you go to the gym like your friend?) or even behaviours such as raised eyebrows or looks of disappointment will create a feeling of failure and poorer body esteem.

Finally, the transmission of body dissatisfaction may relate not only to modelling, the language used or reinforcement but to the dynamic between the parent and child. In the context of eating disorders, families are said to exist in homeostasis, which means that, like a central heating system, they maintain the status quo by constantly making small adjustments. A child may, therefore, develop an eating disorder as a means to readjust the family system and recreate the status quo. In terms of body dissatisfaction, some research indicates that if the mother-daughter relationship is overly enmeshed or limits the daughter's own autonomy, then the daughter may develop body dissatisfaction (10). Therefore, rather than the child's body dissatisfaction being a product of just the mother's own body dissatisfaction or the words used within the family, it may emerge out of the relationships within the family.

Body dissatisfaction is, therefore, common, with many people feeling negative about aspects of their appearance. Whilst there are many possible causes for this, the two key ones are the media through the processes of social comparison and internalisation and the home environment through modelling, language, reinforcement and relationship dynamics.

How can I improve my body image?

Knowing the underlying causes of body dissatisfaction provides clear insights into how to improve body image through learning to be critical of the media, managing your comparison groups, developing positive self-talk and being kind to yourself.

Being critical of the media: The media, in all its forms, bombards us with images of a version of the ideal, whether it be for skin, lips, hair, stomachs, thighs or breasts and chests. Buffering against this first involves realising that it is all fake. The media has every trick available to it, from makeup, lighting, Photoshop and filters to pure AI, which can change any image into something else or just create images out of nothing. It also lies and can tell us that this face cream worked on this person (aged 70 – really?), that this person used this weight loss drug (did they?) and that this person does daily yoga to achieve this body (just yoga?). The first step towards building your own body esteem is to develop a healthy criticism of the media and think about what else has gone into the images you are seeing, and why they have chosen these images for you to see. We developed a brief intervention to teach young women about the tricks of the media, and it seemed to help protect them against the images they were seeing both immediately and also in the longer term (12,13).

Managing your comparison group: The media works by giving us an unrealistic comparison group, encouraging us to make upward comparisons to these images that are neither real nor attainable, which in turn creates a discrepancy between how we see ourselves and how we want to be. A key challenge to this whole process is to manage your comparison group and find more realistic people to set as your norm. Clearly, the easiest way is to come off social media and use your friends. But even if you cannot come off social media, select a comparison group from your own real life that is the same age, same life stage, same body shape, same lifestyle, who you see for real in your life. That way, you can make your comparison group far more realistic and feel better about where you are in your life. Then, also try to find a better social media set of role models out there to focus on. For me, there are now plenty of women my age who are choosing not to have plastic surgery, are going grey and choosing to embrace the ageing process. They are inspiring to me. But each person needs to actively seek out the kinds of people who can help them feel better about themselves.

Developing positive self-talk: We all have scripts in our heads about who we are and how we look that stem from our childhoods, but are embedded by others in our lives as we grow older. For many, these scripts are negative, and we are quick to call ourselves 'useless', lazy', 'fat', 'slow' or 'ugly' because that is what we have heard said about us in the past. To develop a more positive sense of self and reduce any body negativity, these words first need to be identified, then rescripted into something more positive. To identify them, start keeping a diary and every time a word pops into your head, write it down, together with the trigger and the situation you are in. After a week or so, collate these words together and look for patterns. Then try to take perspective and either ask a close friend who is on your side, or be your own friend, and look at each word in turn and in a checklist, replace that word with a more positive one. For example, 'fat' could become 'curvy', 'lazy' could be 'relaxed', or 'slow' could become 'thoughtful'. This way, you can start to build a positive repertoire of self-talk. Next, allow yourself to simply reject them. This has been called the F*** it button, but you can use whatever language you like. But if there are negative words inside your head when you use them, learn to say, 'That's rubbish', 'absolutely not' or learn to blame the person who put them there, 'you not me' and 'how dare you − it's you that is ugly, not me'. That way, you can start to build a new kinder inner voice to start to build a more positive narrative about who you are.

Practice self-compassion: The third strategy that can help to build a more positive relationship with your body is to be kind to yourself and show self-compassion (1,14). The media offers us ideals that are fake and cannot (and should not) be our role models. So be kind to yourself when you see a difference between what you see in the media and how you look. Think − the people I see are fake and AI-generated. If they are not fake, think – the people I see are models and do not have busy jobs or children, friends and family to look after. If they do have children and busy jobs, think – my life is written on my face and body and makes me who I am. I am proud of how I live my life. Further, focus on the positive aspects of your body rather than the negatives. Over the past few years, there has been a shift towards thinking about what bodies can do rather than how they look. Celebrate your body for being strong, able to move well, have children, carry children, run, do yoga, keep a house clean, hug people, etc. Then you can be kinder to yourself if you feel you do not match up to some version of how bodies look, as yours is a body that can do.

In summary

Having a good relationship with your body involves understanding the causes of body dissatisfaction and then protecting yourself against these causes by becoming critical of the media, managing your comparison group, practising positive self-talk and being kind to yourself. That way, we can undo some of the harm done through the media and our childhoods and build a buffer zone between ourselves and any negativity from either inside our heads or the world around us.

To conclude

Eating well as an adult involves developing a good relationship with both food and your body. This involves managing the what, where, when, why and how of what you eat in order to put food back into its box through avoiding emotional and mindless eating and any rebound effects. It also involves minimising body criticism through learning to be critical of the media and using techniques such as positive comparisons, taking perspective and rescripting. All of which has been kind to yourself at its core.

REFERENCES

1. Gilbert, P. (2014). The origins and nature of compassion focused therapy. *British Journal of Clinical Psychology*, 53(1), 6–41.

2. Grogan, S. (2021). *Body Image: Understanding Body Dissatisfaction in Men, Women and Children*, 4th ed. London: Routledge.

3. Ogden, J., and Taylor, C. (2000). Body size evaluation and body dissatisfaction within couples. *International Journal of Health Psychology*, 5, 25–32.

4. Tiggemann, M. (2006). The role of media exposure in adolescent girl's body dissatisfaction and drive for thinness: Prospective results. *Journal of Social and Clinical Psychology*, 25(5), 523–541.

5. Ogden, J., and Mundray, K. (1996). The effect of the media on body satisfaction: The role of gender and size. *European Eating Disorders Review*, 4, 171–182.

6. Groesz, L.M., Levine, M.P., and Murnen, S.K. (2002). The effect of experimental presentation of thin media images on body satisfaction: A meta-analytical review. *International Journal of Eating Disorders*, 31, 1–16.

7. Cash, T.F. (2005). The influence of sociocultural factors on body image: Searching for constructs. *Clinical Psychology: Science and Practice*, 12, 438–442. https://doi.org/10.1093/clipsy.bpi055

8. Thompson, J.K., van den Berg, P., Roehrig, M., Guarda, A.S., and Heinberg, L.S. (2004). The Sociocultural Attitudes Towards Appearance Scale-3 (SATAQ-3): Development and validation. *International Journal of Eating Disorders*, 35, 293–304.

9. Ogden, J., Elias, M., Pletosu, A., Sampang Rai, P., and Zhelyazkova, R. (2024). The relationship between caregivers and daughters' food and body shape scripts: A dyadic analysis. *Appetite*. 2024 Sep 1;200:107560. https://doi.org/10.1016/j.appet.2024.107560

10. Ogden, J., and Steward, J. (2000). The role of the mother daughter relationship in explaining weight concern. *International Journal of Eating Disorders*, 28, 78–83.

11. Brown, R., and Ogden, J. (2004). Children's eating attitudes and behaviour: a study of the modelling and control theories of parental influence. *Health Education Research: Theory and Practice*, 19, 261–271.

12. Ogden, J., and Sherwood, F. (2008). Reducing the impact of media images: An evaluation of the effectiveness of an airbrushing educational intervention on body dissatisfaction. *Health Education*, 108, 489–500.

13. Ogden, J., Smith, L., Nolan, H., Moroney, R., and Lynch, H. (2011). The impact of an educational intervention to protect women against the influence of media images. *Health Education, 111, 412–424.*

14. Gilbert, P. (2010). *The Compassionate Mind: A New Approach to Life's Challenges.* Oakland, CA: New Harbinger Publications. ISBN 9781572248403.

SECTION IV

EATING WELL TO PROMOTE WELLBEING IN LATER LIFE

9

HOW DOES THE ROLE OF FOOD CHANGE IN LATER LIFE?

Eating well is about much more than just nutrition and involves building a good relationship with food. So far, this book has emphasised this in terms of putting food back into its box and managing the when, where, how, and why of eating. For children, this involves building good habits as early as possible, and for adults, this often involves changing unhealthy habits. For many, this also involves trying to eat well in a world pushing us to eat more than we need. As we age, however, the problem seems to reverse, and the key problem of ageing is one of undereating, weight loss, and malnutrition. Eating well as we age is, therefore, often about trying to maintain a healthy weight, avoiding weight loss and having a 'good enough' healthy and balanced diet. This chapter will describe the role of food as we age, with a focus on our physical and mental health as we develop illnesses, become frail or avoid social situations and illustrate how food can also offer a solution to some of the problems ageing brings. It will then address why we tend to eat less as we age due to changes in our biology, social, and psychological lives and our environment. The next chapter will offer solutions to some of these problems.

DOI: 10.4324/9781003600183-15

WHAT IS THE ROLE OF FOOD IN HEALTH AND WELLBEING IN LATER LIFE?

Throughout our lives, food has a key role to play in our physical and mental health. As we grow older, whilst the role of food remains important, it can change as our physical bodies age and our psychological and social lives evolve.

Food and our physical health

Food is key to staying physically well as we age. The ageing process can lead to muscle weakness, which increases the chance of falls if we lose core strength. In turn, falls can often lead to broken hips, arms or collar bones, which can take a while to heal, causing further muscle weakness if a person becomes immobile. Bones also become thinner due to osteoporosis, particularly in women after the menopause, which again can lead to fractures. In addition, our teeth can break and fall out, making it harder to eat, and can cause embarrassment in social situations if a person has gaps and does not wear dentures. Food may not be able to prevent the ageing process, but it can help, and a diet high in protein can help to maintain muscle mass and one high in calcium, through fish or dairy products, can protect our bones and teeth. This can also be helped through supplements such as vitamin C and D, and an intake of lots of fruit and vegetables.

As we age, we can also suffer from urinary incontinence, acid reflux, and constipation or diarrhoea as our muscles loosen and our digestion changes. Again, food is not the magic solution to these changes, but it can help. For example, drinking more water can help with incontinence and constipation; avoiding caffeine, fizzy drinks, and alcohol can help with acid reflux; eating more fruit and vegetables can help with constipation, and a generally healthy diet can help with diarrhoea. Changing the timing of food can also be beneficial, and as we age, people often find it helps to eat more and keep hydrated towards the middle of the day rather than at the end to help with digestion. This can also help with sleep by enabling food to be properly digested before bedtime and reducing the need to get up in the night.

Food is also key to preventing and treating illness. For example, a healthy diet full of fruit and vegetables, high in complex carbohydrates with a moderate amount of protein and fatty foods, but low in sweet foods and those that have been ultra-processed, can protect against many conditions, including heart disease, stroke, diabetes, cancer, and dementia, all of which become increasingly common as we age. Once diagnosed with a health condition, a healthy diet can also be part of the treatment programme. For example, rehabilitation after a stroke or heart attack will involve the recommendation to eat more fruit and vegetables and less fat to reduce the risk of another cardiac event, and type 2 diabetes can be managed by reducing carbohydrates and increasing fruit and vegetable intake. Furthermore, whilst the evidence is poor for the role of diet in the cure of cancer or dementia, there is much evidence that a healthy diet can improve wellbeing and quality of life for those with these conditions (1–3).

Our diet is, therefore, a key part of staying physically well as we age.

Food and our mental health

Food also plays many roles in our mental health and is key to our mood, how we feel about ourselves, the pleasure and fun we get from life and the interactions we have with others. As we age, our relationship with food changes in many ways.

At times, ageing can have a detrimental impact on our ability to eat well, which can, in turn, impact our well-being. For example, throughout our lives, food plays a key part in our social world as we have meals to celebrate birthdays, weddings, religious festivals, and see friends and family. As we age, we may find such social events more problematic if we are tired and need to go to bed earlier than others, are frail and fear falling when we are out, worry about needing the toilet, have to stick to a daily routine in order to manage our medication or simply find it difficult to hear in a group. All these changes can result in someone dropping out of social events and missing out on the pleasure that the food and friendship can bring. Food may also have been a part of our self-identity if we were the person who cooked for others and hosted family get-togethers. Once this time is over, people (particularly women) can feel that they have lost their roles and may not be sure how they fit into their family anymore. Food is also key to how we regulate our emotions, as we use food to boost our mood and treat ourselves. This may become harder to do as we age; if we find it harder to buy food and bring it into the house, it becomes more difficult to go out to meet others to eat with or simply do not get the same rewards from food when we eat alone and find ourselves missing those who are no longer with us.

Food, however, can also be a means of improving wellbeing in later life. Much of life is built around habits and routines that can give our lives structure and meaning, and help the day to pass pleasantly. As children, our day will be built around school, friends, playing, having tea, and bedtime stories. As adults, the structure is often provided by the working day, picking up and feeding children, and seeing friends in the evening. As we age, and many of these responsibilities have passed, our days can feel vague and woolly, as if there is no point. Food is a necessary part of staying alive and involves shopping, preparing, eating and clearing away, and can, therefore, provide a structure and a sense of punctuation. As we age, food can, therefore, offer a boost to mental health by filling time and giving meaning to our day. Food can also be the excuse to have family over (for dinner), to visit family (for dinner), to see friends (for lunch) or to get out of the house and sit in the local café and chat to fellow coffee drinkers and cake eaters. Food is the way into lots of social interactions, even with strangers, which can provide a great lift in wellbeing.

In summary

Food is central to our physical and mental health, and this can change as we grow older. At times, this can come with problems as we develop illnesses, become frail, or avoid social situations. Food, however, can also offer a solution to some of the problems ageing brings and can be a means to avoid illness and stay well, as well as offering structure to our lives and an excuse to meet up with people and chat.

WHY CAN EATING BECOME HARDER AS WE AGE?

The vast majority of books on eating behaviour focus on the problems of overeating in the context of weight gain and obesity. As we age, the key problem is often the opposite – undereating, weight loss, and malnutrition. This section will look at the key biological, social, psychological, and environmental causes behind this change.

Changes to our biology

As we age, there are many changes in our biology that can result in undereating. First, we often become less active and lose muscle mass, and as a result, our body may simply feel less hungry. This can result in simply forgetting to eat at all or just getting full quicker when we start to eat. We are also more likely to have health conditions, which can make eating more difficult. For example, diabetes and dementia can directly impact upon our desire to eat by changing our ability to detect and respond to hunger signals; conditions such as heart disease, dementia, stroke, COPD, or Parkinson's can create muscle weakness or coordination problems, which make it more difficult to actually eat and many medications for many conditions can change our taste preferences and make food less enjoyable. Furthermore, fear of incontinence can make people anxious about drinking, which, in turn, can trigger constipation, again impacting their appetite. Frailty is common as we age and can create muscle weakness and a fear of falling, making any activity, including shopping, cooking, and eating, not only more tiring but also more worrying. People can also lose their ability to see or hear, which can make them become more socially isolated as they feel uncomfortable in company. This can mean they avoid social situations with others, which can result in them staying at home rather than eating with friends and family. Finally, sleep patterns can become more problematic as we age, with people feeling more tired, needing to go to bed earlier, or not being able to sleep as long. This can disrupt meal patterns and make people avoid social events if they go on later into the evening. Together, all these factors can result in weight loss and malnutrition.

Changes to our social lives

Food is a key part of how we socially interact with others and has a role to play in many family, friendship, religious, and cultural celebrations. It is also at the heart of chatting with friends and popping out for a coffee. As we age, this can be sustained if families are nearby or if we become members of community groups through religion, charities, sport or social clubs. But as families become more disparate and children and grandchildren move away, local community groups close due to lack of funding and getting out and about gets harder when people stop driving or struggle with mobility; interacting with others becomes more of an effort and any social eating is reduced.

As people age, they also often end up living alone. This can have a huge impact on eating, as shopping for food, cooking and eating meals play such a pivotal role in our home lives. When we are, therefore, left alone, it can become difficult to find the motivation to cook a proper meal, and people often resort to ready meals, snacking or just having things on toast. Once living alone, there is no one else to remind us to eat, make us dinner, or pop to the shops for some cake. Food intake is, therefore, reduced, and eating can become a chore.

Furthermore, whilst the modern world is set up for eating at home and not cooking through using home deliveries, this may not be accessible to older people who may well not be computer literate and may find it an anathema to shop online, have strangers deliver food, or to eat food prepared by others in ways that are not familiar to them.

Changes to our psychology

This book has emphasised how food is often used as a key part of emotional regulation and has highlighted how we learn from childhood to use food as treats and rewards in our daily lives. As we age, this association between food and our mood can also change. For many, there will always be the pick-me-up of a cake mid-afternoon or a biscuit with a cup of tea. But as shopping, cooking, and eating become more problematic, people may turn to other means to manage their mood, such as watching TV, doing puzzles, or listening to the radio – all of which are less effort, more sedentary and less tiring. Further, many will also develop a lower mood if their efforts at emotional regulation become less effective. This, in turn, can all lead to eating less.

Food is also a key part of how we communicate and can be a form of self-expression and a statement of our identity. As we age, this can also change. For many, being a cook may remain key if they cook for their families and treat their grandchildren to homemade cakes and biscuits. But for some, this becomes harder if families are dispersed, if people are living alone, and if there is no one there to benefit from food as a treat, a reward or as a show of love. Again, food intake can be reduced.

Eating is also a habit, and over the course of our lives, we learn to associate food with certain times of day, specific people and places, our routines, such as doing a crossword or watching TV, and it becomes key to how we punctuate our lives. As we age, many of these habits are broken as we change who we live with, where we live, and what activities we can do. We can therefore no longer rely on eating as a response to these triggers in our world, which can take away many of the prompts to eat in our daily lives.

A reduction in both emotional eating and eating as a form of communication, therefore, leads to undereating. Further, as our habits are broken, many of the prompts to eat vanish from our lives. Together, these can lead to malnutrition.

Changes to our environment

One of the key triggers to eating is our food environment, and for many, this can lead to mindless eating as food is just there. For children and adults, this can often lead to overeating, and we often encourage people to eat more mindfully so that they are aware of what they are eating and can make better choices. But as we age, our food environment changes, which can lead to undereating. Frailty and illness can mean that people go out less and are, less exposed to food in cafes, the cinema, or around a friend's house. If they shop less due to ill health or living alone, their home environment can also become depleted of food triggers if their fridge and cupboards are only rarely restocked. And when people cook for one rather than their partner or family, they are more likely to cook smaller portions or eat pre-packed ready meals, leaving no leftovers to snack on later. As we age, we are exposed to fewer food triggers, making it harder to eat mindlessly. And, ironically, as we age, more mindless eating can become a good thing.

In summary

We, eat less as we age due to our biology, social world, psychology, and environment, which can remove the triggers to eat for social interaction, emotional regulation, communication and mindless eating. We, therefore, need some strategies to make sure we can reverse these effects and help everyone eat well into their older age.

To conclude

Ageing brings with it changes to our physical bodies and can result in frailty or illness. Furthermore, we can become isolated or lonely. Together, all these changes can result in undereating, weight loss, and malnutrition. Food cannot solve all the problems of physical ageing, but it can help, and by eating well, some of the symptoms of ageing can be delayed; some illnesses can be managed, and some even prevented. Likewise, food can also provide an excuse to facilitate social interactions with friends, family, and even strangers and can offer a way to structure and punctuate our daily lives. Together, whilst ageing does have many negative consequences and can result in undereating, food can also be key to maintaining our sense of wellbeing.

REFERENCES

1. Castro-Espin, C., and Agudo, A. (2022). The role of diet in prognosis among cancer survivors: A systematic review and meta-analysis of dietary patterns and diet interventions. *Nutrients*, 14(2), 348. doi:10.3390/nu14020348. PMID: 35057525; PMCID: PMC8779048.
2. WHO (2020). Healthy diet. www.who.int/news-room/fact-sheets/detail/healthy-diet (accessed July 2, 2025).
3. WHO (2003). Diet, nutrition and the prevention of chronic diseases: Report of a Joint WHO/FAO Expert Consultation. WHO Technical Report Series, No. 916. Geneva: World Health Organization.

10

HOW CAN WE ENSURE PEOPLE EAT WELL AS THEY AGE?

The main problem with ageing is one of undereating and weight loss, which can come with frailty and illness. This chapter will explore how we can look after ourselves as we age by keeping an eye on our weight, planning regular, smaller meals, making the most of social and mindless eating whenever we can, taking supplements, and being kind to ourselves by eating what we like and cooking food that is 'good enough'. It will then offer some tips for helping others to eat well when they are either living independently or in residential care. It highlights the importance of making eating as easy, social and mindless as possible and highlighting that something is often better than nothing. This can help maximise the impact of food on physical health and also be a useful tool to improve wellbeing through encouraging social interaction, promoting a sense of independence and providing a structure to the day.

HOW CAN WE CARE FOR OURSELVES AS WE AGE?

Many people can undereat and lose weight as they age due to changes in their biology, social worlds, psychology and environment. Making

DOI: 10.4324/9781003600183-16

sure we still eat enough of the right kinds of foods as we age is, therefore, key to staying well and involves finding other ways to build eating into our daily lives. Here are some tips for making food a core part of self-care.

Be aware of your body weight

The focus on body weight, shape, and size can be damaging to children and adults. But as we age, it is a good idea to be aware of any unintended weight loss. Therefore, watch for signs that your clothes or jewellery are becoming looser, listen if your friends or family tell you that you are losing weight and ask the doctor to weigh you whenever you have an appointment. Even buy some bathroom scales so that you can watch your weight every month to check for any decline, but do not do this if you have any history of weight concern or disordered eating. As we age, we lose muscle, which we need for strength and mobility. We also need a bit more padding if we fall and to keep us warm. Therefore, after about age 70, it is rare that weight loss is a good thing. I have known several women who have struggled with being overweight all their lives and who have welcomed their weight loss in older age. This has seemed very close to an eating disorder, as they have encouraged the newfound ability to miss meals and have enjoyed being the coveted skinnier version of themselves. So be aware of your weight; do not revel in any weight loss, and if you experience unintended weight loss, go to your doctor to check for any underlying causes, and then think about ways to increase your food intake.

Build new habits

Most of this book has emphasised the benefits of eating three meals a day and avoiding snacking. As we age, it is sometimes overwhelming to have a large portion of food placed in front of us. It can also seem like a long time between meals when we live alone, and the day is lonely. As we age, it is better to have six smaller meals a day rather than three and to build these into our daily routine. So have breakfast, a mid-morning snack, lunch, mid-afternoon snack, dinner and then an evening snack to finish off the day. Do not skip meals and try to eat these at a table or on a specific chair so that you can start to build up new habits triggered by seeing this table or that chair.

Plan what to eat

It is good to have ingredients as well as meals in the cupboard so that you can eat regularly every day. This is helped through planning what and when you are going to eat, making a shopping list, and then planning when you are going to the shops. If you prefer to go to the local shop regularly, then this trip can become part of your daily routine. This is also a good way to get out and to see people for a chat. If you prefer to do a weekly shop, then try to plan this alongside a coffee with a friend to make it a sociable experience.

Eat socially

Most of us eat more when we are with others – a process of social facilitation. Try to build eating into your social events, whether it is having a friend round for coffee (and a biscuit) or meeting family for a Sunday lunch at a pub. Also, use your friends and family to help you eat well and let them know you are concerned about losing weight, so they can bring food when they visit or take you out with them for visits to the garden centre or art gallery (and café).

Eat mindlessly

Mindless eating is not great in a world full of food, but as we age, we can use mindless eating to help us stay well. Make food easily available and visible in your home by having bowls of fruit or nuts around so you can pick while you are watching TV or listening to the radio. Take food into the car so you can snack whilst driving and settle on the sofa with some fruit or cake at the end of the day to watch a film. For most of our lives, this is often discouraged, but as we age, eating something is often better than nothing, and simply having it available is a good way to make sure we eat more than our bodies might be telling us to.

Take supplements

Ideally, we would get all the nutrition we need from eating well. But given the changes in older age, this is not always possible, so supplements can be a good way to make sure we have the right nutrients in our diet. The shops have several age-appropriate vitamin and mineral packs which you can get from the pharmacist. But in addition, try to up your intake in other ways, such as having full-fat milky drinks, buying fortified bread or cereals, adding protein powder to soups and having smoothies to drink full of fruit and vegetables. Then build these into your daily routine so you have a smoothie for breakfast and a milky drink before bed.

Eat what you like

As we age, our tastes change, and people can find they like sweeter foods, spicier foods, or softer foods, which require less effort to eat. From a nutrition perspective, we should always eat a balanced diet full of fruit and vegetables, moderate in complex carbohydrates, moderate in protein and fatty foods, and low in sweet foods. As we age, this is still the case, but the priorities can change. If a person is becoming underweight or malnourished, then they just need to eat more. If they have been ill and lost weight, then they just need to gain some weight. And if they have lost their appetite through illness or medication, they need to be tempted back into eating with whatever works for them. If this is the case, then eat whatever you fancy. If you want cake, have some, but try to have a fruit cake or sponge with raspberries on it. If you want a pudding, have a fruit crumble with custard. If you want ice cream, then have some blueberries with it if you can. And if you want lasagne for breakfast and toast for your dinner, then that is fine. Being well is the goal, so whatever gets you to this goal is fine.

Make it easy for yourself

The world is full of cookery programmes with chefs preparing amazing meals. Whilst great to watch, these have managed to up our expectations of what food is and what we should be eating, whilst, at the same time, trapping people on their sofa as they order takeaways. As we get older, we need to eat well, and this does not mean eating like a chef. It means eating in a way that is good enough to keep you well. So, shop, cook, and eat in ways that make it easy for yourself. It is, therefore, fine to have ready meals sometimes, but try to have vegetables on the side. When you cook, try to cook more than you need so you can freeze a portion and have it another day. Roll over meals to reduce cooking time – sausage and mash can become the mash of cottage pie if you cook enough, and roast chicken leftovers can become chicken curry or chicken and bacon pasta. And sometimes, a simple jacket potato with cheese and salad or beans on toast can be good enough. Do not skip meals. But do not feel that every meal has to be a cookery feast (do have a look at the recipes at the end of this book!).

In summary

Eating well as we age often involves trying to eat even when our bodies are not telling us to. We, therefore, need to try to build new habits by planning regular, smaller meals, making the most of social and mindless eating whenever we can, taking supplements and wedging in food and being kind to ourselves by eating what we like and cooking food that is good enough to be eaten by us, not by a TV chef.

HOW CAN WE CARE FOR OTHERS AS THEY AGE?

As people age, they can start to lose independence and need different degrees of looking after by others. This may involve having family members pop round more often to provide some degree of support in their own home, having formal carers either living in or paying regular visits, moving into supported accommodation where many aspects of independence are maintained or moving into a form of residential care where responsibilities for many aspects of self-care are taken on by the staff. Food plays a central role in self-care. It also plays a role in caring for others. This section will provide some tips for how to encourage someone else you are caring for to eat well, either whilst they are living independently or when delivering residential care.

HOW DO I CARE FOR SOMEONE LIVING INDEPENDENTLY?

Whether it is a neighbour, parent, friend, or sibling, many of us offer unofficial care to others as they age that involves food in some way. Here are some tips to help someone else eat well as they age.

Make it easy for them

Eating well involves shopping, preparing, eating, and clearing up. As we age, this can become tiring and increasingly difficult if we are frightened of falling, can no longer drive, have trouble carrying heavy bags, or are losing our vision. If you are helping someone stay well, then try to make this process as easy as possible for them – plan their meals with them, bring their shopping in, make their lunch and offer to do the washing up. Also suggest some easier meals that are still nutritious, such as jacket potatoes (in the microwave), beans and salad; fish fingers, chips and peas; sausages and mash and peas;

and even ready meals such as fish pie or lasagne that are not over-processed. Food does not have to be complicated or perfect. But encourage them NOT to skip meals and emphasise that food can be kept simple. Something is better than nothing.

A little and often

As people age, they sometimes cannot manage larger meals as they feel full quickly. It is therefore better to encourage them to eat a little and often. This could take the format of six smaller meals a day, with three meals interspaced with larger snacks. So, if you help them with their shopping, make sure they have plenty of ingredients to make frequent eating easier. If you do some of their cooking, make several meals at a time so they have something prepared for later, and if they have a dishwasher, offer to unpack it every other day to cut out the washing up.

Make it social

We eat more when we are with others, and eating with others can be a great source of social interaction. Try to sit with someone when they are eating for a chat, or even better, eat your meal with them. That way, you can make sure they are eating and encourage them to eat more. Sometimes, take them out to a café to be with other people eating and build in snacks to your outings to garden centres, museums or art galleries.

Encourage mindless eating

We can only eat food if it is there, so make sure they have food in the house, and then make it visible and available by having bowls of nuts or fruit on the table or the biscuit tin near the kettle. If you have prepared their meal, leave it out so they will not forget to have it or leave a meal plan stuck to the fridge so they can see what meals to have and when.

Make it fun

Eating should be fun, and by having fun, we are more likely to eat again. If they like cooking, encourage them to make you scones or cakes and express your pleasure when you get them. Or ask them to make you your favourite tea and then sit with them whilst you drink it. And chat whilst you eat, so they can eat more without thinking. If they do not like cooking, then do it for them when you can, or set up a delivery system and let them eat what they fancy. Food should be healthyish, but if they enjoy it, that's mostly better than nothing.

Reward 'good behaviour'

Eating well as we age is about trying to maintain a healthy weight, avoiding weight loss and having a good enough, healthy and balanced diet, and, as with all behaviours, this is more likely to happen if it is rewarded. But the aim is also to offer this reward in a way that does no harm. So if the aim is to help someone regain weight, given the current preoccupation with being thin, it is better to say, 'You do look well', 'You are looking healthier', 'You have got some of your colour back' or 'You are looking stronger by the day' than 'well done you have put on weight' or 'you have got a bit fatter since I last saw you'. Weight bias exists all the way through our lives, and even very thin, underweight people do not want to hear that they are fatter. Likewise, if the goal is to get someone to eat more it is better to say, 'That's great, you did enjoy that', 'That will do you good' or 'It's lovely to see you getting your appetite back' rather than, 'Gosh, you wolfed that down' or 'You're like a bottomless pit'. Rewarding weight gain and eating more will make it continue, but do it in ways that are not harmful and do not backfire.

Focus on the immediate benefits

Eating well in older age can be about preventing illness, treating illness and living longer. But these are longer-term goals, and our behaviour is much more likely to be impacted by more immediate benefits. So, if you are encouraging someone to eat well, eat more or gain weight, focus on short-term outcomes such as feeling stronger, having more energy, being able to sleep better, having better skin, having stronger hair, having a better colour, being less likely to fall and being able to become more independent. These are within reach and attainable and are much more likely to encourage eating well than goals in the future.

In summary

Helping someone else to eat well as they age is about making it as easy, sociable, and fun as possible, encouraging regular, smaller meals and emphasising that something is better than nothing and using words of praise that avoid doing any harm.

HOW DO I CARE FOR SOMEONE LIVING IN RESIDENTIAL CARE?

There are many types of residential care homes which vary hugely in terms of the needs of the residents, the available finances, and the structure of the building being used. But whatever the situation, there are some key principles for encouraging older people to eat well and for using food to support their wellbeing and happiness.

How can I encourage people to eat well?

Below are some tips to help people eat well when they are living in residential care.

Maintain a sense of independence

Even when people are living in care, most still want to feel some sense of independence. This can be achieved in ways that can also encourage people to eat well such as giving them a choice of food through a daily menu, making sure there is some variety of food so there is something for everyone, having eating areas that are outside of the bedrooms and separate to other social areas, encouraging people not to eat in their rooms, and making the eating areas feel as much like a comfortable eating space as possible.

Use social interaction

Given that we tend to eat more when we eat with others, encouraging social eating can also encourage people to eat more. This can be achieved in residential care by having social tables for people to eat at, allowing people to choose who they sit with, encouraging people to include new people in their eating groups, giving people time to eat slowly if they need to and encouraging people to stay at the table until everyone has finished. It can also be achieved by having regular breaks throughout the day for tea and biscuits, and coffee and cake to encourage people into the social spaces. For those residents who cannot leave their rooms, it is also best to encourage them to eat socially where possible. This can involve asking family or friends to stay for mealtimes, having carers sit with residents where possible or even pairing up more able with less able residents and asking them to help out by sitting with those who need to remain in their rooms. It can also help if staff members have their meals in the same room as the clients and are seen to enjoy what they are eating. Any form of social interaction can encourage people to eat well.

Use rewards

Eating well can also be encouraged through rewards. This can simply be through conversations with comments such as 'You have done well' and 'Well done for trying that', or through encouragement, such as 'Just try to have a bit more', 'It will help build up your strength' and 'It's so nice to see you getting your appetite back'.

Use mindless eating

Mindless eating can also be a useful tool in care homes, and people will eat food if it is there. So, it can help to have bowls of crisps or fruit around in the common areas to help people snack, to make sure that drinks come with biscuits and that there is bread and butter on the table before a meal is served.

How can food be used to improve wellbeing?

Much as food is key to staying physically well, and we need to encourage people to eat well, food is also a useful tool to improve wellbeing.

Encouraging social interaction

When in residential care, people can become isolated and lonely and trapped in their rooms due to feelings of tiredness, frailty, fear of falling, failing sight or hearing, muscle weakness, or just getting out of practice for how to interact with others. Food is a great way to encourage people out of their rooms and to interact with others, either through offering snacks in the lounge, meals in the dining room, or having activities that are rewarded with food – bingo and cake, music and biscuits, stretching and snacks, may all add the extra incentive to get people taking part. Food is also a great way to make new friends as it offers a topic of conversation about what we like to eat or do not, and whether the chef is up to our standards or not. Preparing food can also be a fun and social activity, which takes the stress out of the topic of conversation, whilst creating something to be shared later.

Regulating emotions

Food can also be a means to help people manage their emotions. As we age, many of our sources of pleasure can disappear as we lose friends and partners, are no longer able to play sport or go to the theatre and may miss the garden or the pet we have given up to come into residential care. Food can provide a way to boost and manage our mood through giving the day a structure and making it pass easily, by reminding us of our childhoods and happier times, through bringing back memories of fish and chips of the beach or trifle for Sunday dinner, by helping us connect with our culture even if we are no longer living in our country of birth, by feeling cared for by others and by enabling us to care for others by helping the person in the next room finish their meal. Together, food is so embedded with meaning that it can help bring back positive feelings and generate new ones.

Providing structure and rhythm

Life in a care home can become dull and boring as so many parts of daily life can be stripped away, leaving a TV as the last vestige of amusement. Food is not only good for getting people together and helping with mood; it also offers a structure to the day and a way to punctuate time. This gives the day a rhythm and can make an empty day feel busy and lively if one meal is always finishing as the next is being prepared and looked forward to.

Rebuilding a sense of self

Much of our sense of self can start to wane as we age, particularly when we give up our independence and move into residential care. Food is a core part of our sense of identity and reflects who we are in terms of our culture, our relationships, our interests and our history. Food can therefore be used to help rebuild our sense of self, even when many aspects of our lives have changed. Having a menu to choose what to eat can give us a sense of autonomy; eating with friends can remind us that we are interesting and fun; having family in to join us for a meal can make us feel loved; being helped to eat when we are no longer able to do so on our own make us feel important and choosing a treat from our childhoods can make us feel young again.

In summary

Food is key to caring for someone in residential care. Whilst there may be a tendency to eat less and lose weight as we age, strategies can be used in residential care to encourage eating well through giving people choice and variety of foods, using social interaction to encourage social eating, offering praise for eating well and providing opportunities for mindless eating. But food is much more than just about nutrition and offers a useful tool to improve wellbeing through tempting people out of their rooms to interact with others, giving them a boost to their mood, providing a structure to the day and helping them re-find their sense of self.

To conclude

Much of childhood and adulthood is about building healthy eating habits and learning to manage a food environment designed to make us overeat. As we age, the problem is often reversed and becomes one of undereating, weight loss, and even malnutrition. This chapter has explored how we can look after ourselves as we age through becoming aware of changes in our body weight, eating more regularly, maximising the impact of social and mindless eating, and making it easy for ourselves by having a 'good enough' principle and eating what we like. This chapter has also explored how to help others eat well. Whether they are living independently or are in residential care, eating well still involves using social and mindless eating to their benefit, but also adding in rewards and making food fun. But food is also core to wellbeing and can be a useful tool to alleviate boredom, boost mood, encourage friendships and help rebuild a sense of self, particularly when living in a care setting, when people can become isolated and stuck in their rooms.

CONCLUDING COMMENTS

Eating well is about so much more than nutrition and can go wrong in many ways. This book has outlined what it means to eat well and develop a good relationship with food at every age to maximise both our physical health and wellbeing.

Childhood is a time when key eating habits are developed. This book has described the three pillars of good food parenting as being a good role model, saying the right things, and managing one's environment. It has then illustrated how these can offer useful solutions to many problems faced as children grow up, whether it be not wanting to eat a healthy diet, eating too much or too little, developing poor body image, or spending too much time just sitting.

Adulthood is often a time when poor habits need to be unlearned and when the world around us seems designed to make us overeat or eat the wrong foods, and when food and our body size can become a source of anxiety. This book has offered many solutions to changing what we eat, either for weight loss or just to be healthier – but in ways that avoid harm and do not make things worse. It has also focused on just feeling good about yourself and being kind – aim high, but let yourself off when things do not quite work out.

As we age into older life, things often change, and the problem can be one of undereating, weight loss, and malnutrition. Food is part of managing our physical health and can help buffer against some of the changes brought by ageing. But food can also help with wellbeing as it offers a source of pleasure, structure, and a useful excuse for spending time with friends and family. As we age, however, our bodies often seem to tell us to eat less than we need. This

DOI: 10.4324/9781003600183-17

chapter has, therefore, described useful strategies to make sure we eat well as we age and can care for others, whether they are living independently or in residential care.

Throughout this book, I have drawn upon a wealth of psychological research and theory, but kept references to a minimum. If you want to read more, do have a look at the reference list or the further reading list.

I have also added some recipes at the end compiled by me and my friends whilst our children were still at home, which were healthy enough and kept us sane.

FINAL WORDS

I have spent 38 years researching eating behaviour. Along the way, I have seen friends struggle with eating disorders where food has become ridden with anxiety and guilt. I have met many patients living with obesity who struggle to lose weight, and when they do, they struggle to keep it off. And I have heard so many people say they feel fat, do not like their bottom, stomach, legs, or chest and just find food difficult. I have watched friends hover around their children, bribing them with pudding to get them to eat their vegetables, and I have heard them say that they are too busy or tired to cook, but then feel guilty for ordering a takeaway. And I have seen elderly men and women in care homes left on their own to eat mush when they can hardly hold their heads up. And all the while, I have watched as the food industry has often done its very best to make it very hard to eat well.

And in my own life, I have tried to use at least some of what I have learnt with my own children and my fairly large extended family. I have said and done many things along the way that were not great, and I have developed a very strong, good enough principle. This book is my attempt to put that research into practice and make it available to the real world of people just trying to do a good job.

The modern world makes it very easy to gain weight, hard to stay healthy and easy to develop a difficult relationship with food. I hope that this book has offered some useful ways to manage this without making food into a problem. Feeding ourselves with other unhealthy foods is not great. But having a problem with food for the rest of our lives is far, far worse

SOME RECIPES FOR YOU!

I hope it is now clear I am not a chef, nor a nutritionist, nor a dietician. Nor do I really like cooking! But over the years, I have asked my friends for advice on what to cook that is easy and healthy that we can all eat together. Here are some simple meals we have come up with that work when time is short and life is busy. I have classified them in terms of preparation time (effort) AND cooking time (fridge to table), as some meals require you to be in the kitchen the whole time, whilst others involve putting things on to cook, then having time to do something else. You can mix and match the different meals, but each meal should have a base of carbohydrate (bread/pasta/potato/rice) and at least two vegetables. If you do not eat meat, then you can substitute the meat for another source of protein, such as soya-based sausages, mince or pulses. I have described the quantities for a family of two adults and two children who eat almost the same amount as adults. And my top tips:

1. Get a decent pair of kitchen scissors for cutting meat and fish
2. Put the oven and/or kettle on before you start
3. Keep grated cheese in the fridge, ready to go

1. SAUSAGES, MASH AND PEAS (AND ONION GRAVY)

Time: Fridge to table: 1 hour
        Effort: 15 minutes

Ingredients:
3 sausages per person
2 big potatoes per person
Frozen peas
1 onion (for onion gravy – optional)

Preparation
Put oven on (190°C)
Put the kettle on
Place sausages on a tray in the oven for 50 mins (defrost in the microwave first if frozen)
After 40 minutes....
Chop up potatoes into small cubes
Boil potatoes for 15 mins
Place peas and beans in a bowl in the microwave and heat for 8 mins
Strain potatoes, add a splash of milk, a nob of butter and mash up
Chop the onion lengthways and fry with a splash of oil until a bit burnt, add water

Serve....

2. SAUSAGES, POTATO WEDGES AND VEGETABLES

Time: Fridge to table: 1 hour
Effort: 10 minutes

Ingredients
3 sausages per person
3 potatoes per person
Frozen vegetables (peas/beans/broccoli/cauliflower/spinach?)

Procedure
Put oven on (190°C)
Place sausages on a tray in the oven for 50 mins (defrost first in the microwave if frozen)
Slice potatoes longwise into wedges
Place wedges into freezer bag, drizzle in a splash of oil, shake bag a bit
Place wedges on a tray in the oven, turn after 20 mins
Wait 40 mins ….
Cook frozen veg in microwave for 8 mins.

Serve …

3. SAUSAGE CASSEROLE

Time: Fridge to table: 1 hour
Effort: 20 minutes

Ingredients
3 sausages per person
1 onion
I tin of chopped tomatoes
1 tin of beans
Tobasco/Worcester sauce
Frozen vegetables (peas/broccoli/cauliflower)
Can be served with mash or wedges

Procedure
Put oven on (190°C)
Chop the onion into small pieces and fry it with a splash of oil
Add sausages until browned
Transfer to an oven dish with a lid
Add tinned tomatoes, a tin of beans and tobasco / Worcester sauce
Place in the oven for 40 minutes
Wait 30 minutes
Cook frozen vegetables in the microwave for 8 mins

Serve....

4. CHICKEN, BACON, MUSHROOMS AND RICE

Time: Fridge to table: 30 minutes
      Effort: 30 minutes

Ingredients
1 large chicken breast per person
1 bacon slice per person
5 mushrooms
60g brown rice per person
Rosemary and garlic for flavour
Large tablespoon of crème fraiche for the sauce
Frozen beans

Procedure
Put the kettle on
Put rice into a saucepan and boil for 30 minutes
Chop bacon and chicken into bite-sized pieces and fry with a splash of oil
Add garlic
After 20 minutes, add sliced mushrooms
Add rosemary
Heat beans in the microwave for 8 mins
Add crème fraîche to chicken
Drain rice

Serve …

5: LEMON CHICKEN AND RICE

Time: Fridge to table: 30 minutes
          Effort: 20 minutes

Ingredients
1 large chicken breast per person
A dessertspoon of flour
Lemon juice
60 g brown rice per person
Frozen vegetables (peas, beans, broccoli, cauliflower)

Procedure
Put the kettle on
Put rice in a saucepan and boil for 30 minutes
Slice chicken into bite-sized pieces
Put flour on a plate
Roll chicken pieces in flour and shallow fry with a splash of oil
Squirt lemon over chicken
Cook until lightly browned (20 minutes)
Heat vegetables in the microwave
Drain rice

Serve....

5. CHICKEN KEBABS AND CHEESY POTATOES

Time: Fridge to table: 20 minutes
     Effort: 20 minutes

Ingredients
1 big potato per person
1 large chicken breast per person
1 red pepper
Kebab sticks
Grated cheese
Vegetables (peas, beans, broccoli, cauliflower, spinach)

Procedure
Place potatoes in the microwave for 10 mins (until cooked)
Put the grill on
Slice the chicken into 4 pieces each
Chop pepper into chunks
Thread chicken and pepper onto sticks
Place under grill (not too high) for 10 minutes, turning now and again
Slice potatoes in half, lengthwise
Scoop out the middle of each, leaving skins intact and place in a bowl.
Add grated cheese and mix up
Scoop potato mix back into potato skins, drag fork over top
Place under the grill for 5 minutes until brown
Cook vegetables in the microwave

Serve ...

6. SALMON AND RICE

Time: Fridge to table: 30 minutes
       Effort: 10 minutes

Ingredients
1 salmon fillet per person
Lemon juice
60 g brown rice per person
Vegetables (peas, beans, broccoli, cauliflower)

Procedure
Put oven on (190°C)
Put the kettle on
Add rice to water and boil for 30 minutes
Place salmon fillets on an oven tray and squirt lemon juice on top
(defrost in microwave first if frozen)
Place salmon in the oven for 25 minutes.
Heat vegetables in the microwave for 8 minutes.

Serve...

7. CHILLI AND RICE

Time: Fridge to table: 30 minutes
        Effort: 30 minutes

Ingredients
1 small bag of lamb mince
1 onion
1 clove garlic
1 tin chopped tomatoes
5 mushrooms
1 tin of kidney beans
Tobacco/Worcester sauce/Teaspoon of chopped chilli
60 g brown rice per person
Frozen vegetables (beans, peas, broccoli, cauliflower)

Procedure
Put the kettle on
Place rice in a saucepan and boil for 30 minutes
Chop the onion and shallow fry it with a splash of oil
Add garlic
Add mince (if frozen, that is fine)
Stir until the mince is brown
Add chilli, tobacco, Worcester sauce, tomatoes, kidney beans, sliced mushrooms
Place on the lid and cook on low heat for 20 minutes
Heat vegetables in the microwave
Drain rice

Serve....

8. SALMON PASTA

Time: Fridge to table 20 minutes
Effort: 20 minutes

Ingredients
1 large onion
1 salmon fillet per person
A teaspoon of chopped chilli (optional)
Crème fraîche
75 g brown pasta per person
Frozen vegetables (peas, beans, broccoli, cauliflower)

Procedure
Put the kettle on
Chop the onion into small pieces
Shallow fry the onion in a splash of oil until soft
Chop salmon into bite-sized pieces and onions (defrost in microwave if frozen and cut off skin)
Stir until cooked and mash up a bit with a spoon (20 minutes)
Add chilli (optional)
Place the pasta in a pan and boil for 10 minutes
Heat vegetables in microwave (8 minutes)
Add crème fraîche to salmon
Drain pasta
Mix up pasta and salmon

Serve...

8. PASTA PESTO

Time: Fridge to table 15 mins (10 if you have a quick boil kettle)
 Effort: 10 mins

Ingredients
75g brown pasta per person
Jar of green pesto sauce
Salad:
Peppers, cucumber, olives, chopped carrots, lettuce and tomatoes

Procedure
Put the kettle on
Boil pasta in a pan for 10 minutes
Chop salad vegetables and place in a bowl
Drain pasta
Stir 5 teaspoons of pesto into the pasta.

Serve....

9. BACON PASTA

Time: Fridge to table: 15 minutes (10 if you have a quick boil kettle)
Effort: 10 minutes

Ingredients
75 g brown pasta per person
2 slices of unsmoked bacon per person
Grated cheese
Pine nuts (optional)
Salad:
Peppers, cucumber, olives, chopped carrots, lettuce and tomatoes

Procedure
Put the kettle on
Place pasta in a saucepan and boil for 10 minutes
Chop bacon and dry fry for 5 minutes
Add pine nuts (optional)
Chop up salad vegetables and place in a bowl
Drain pasta
Add pasta to bacon, add grated cheese, place on the heat and stir until cheese has melted

Serve....

10. SEAFOOD PASTA

Time: Fridge to table: 30 minutes
Effort: 10 minutes

Ingredients
75 g brown pasta per person
1 bag of frozen seafood mix (squid, mussels, cockles, etc.)
1 onion
1 tin of chopped tomatoes
Tobasco/Worcester sauce/teaspoon of chopped chilli (optional)
Salad:
Peppers, cucumber, olives, chopped carrots, lettuce and tomatoes

Procedure
Put the kettle on
Chop the onion into small pieces
Fry the onion in a splash of oil until soft
Add tinned tomatoes
Add frozen seafood (does not need defrosting)
Add Tobasco/Worcester sauce/chilli (optional)
Stir, then add the lid and leave to simmer for 20 minutes
Chop salad vegetables and place in a bowl
Place the pasta into the pot and boil for 10 minutes
Drain pasta

Serve...

10. SPAGHETTI BOLOGNESE

Time: Fridge to table: 30 minutes
Effort: 30 minutes

Ingredients
1 small bag of lamb mince
1 onion
1 clove garlic
1 tin chopped tomatoes
5 mushrooms
Tobasco/Worcester sauce/Teaspoon of chopped chilli (optional)
75 g brown pasta per person
Frozen vegetables (beans, peas, broccoli, cauliflower)

Procedure
Chop the onion and shallow fry it with a splash of oil
Add garlic
Add mince (if frozen, that is fine)
Stir until the mince is brown
Add chilli, tobasco, Worcester sauce, tomatoes, sliced mushrooms
Place on the lid and cook on low heat for 20 minutes
Place the pasta in a pot and boil for 10 minutes
Heat vegetables in the microwave (8 minutes).
Drain pasta

Serve ...

11. MEATBALL PASTA

Time: Fridge to table 15 minutes
Effort: 15 minutes

Ingredients
Swedish meatballs (already cooked – 8 per person)
1 onion
1 tin of chopped tomatoes
5 mushrooms
Tobasco/Worcester sauce/teaspoon of chopped chilli (optional)
75 g brown pasta per person
Grated cheese
Salad (peppers, cucumber, olives, chopped carrots, lettuce, tomatoes)

Procedure
Put the kettle on
Place the meatballs in a bowl and cook in the microwave for 10 minutes
Place the pasta in the pot and boil for 10 minutes
Chop the onion and shallow fry it with a splash of oil
Add tomatoes
Add Tobacco/Worcester sauce/chilli (optional)
Chop the salad vegetables and place them in a bowl.
Drain the pasta
Mix the meatballs and tomato sauce.

Serve... add grated cheese at the table

11. LEEK AND BACON PASTA

Time: Fridge to table 20 minutes
Effort: 20 minutes

Ingredients
1 leek per person
2 slices of bacon per person
5 mushrooms
Pine nuts (optional)
Grated cheese (cheddar or stilton)
75 g brown pasta per person
Salad (Peppers, cucumber, olives, chopped carrots, lettuce, tomatoes)

Procedure
Put the kettle on
Slice the leeks and wash them in a sieve
Slice bacon and shallow fry leeks with sliced bacon and a splash of oil
Add pine nuts (optional)
Place pasta in pot and boil for 10 minutes
Chop the salad vegetables and place them in a bowl
Drain the pasta
Add pasta to the leeks, add grated cheese and stir until the cheese has melted.

Serve.....

12. STUFFED PASTA

Time: Fridge to table: 10 minutes
      Effort: 10 minutes

Ingredients
Fresh stuffed pasta (100 g per person)
Salad: Peppers, cucumber, olives, chopped carrots, lettuce, tomatoes
Grated cheese

Procedure
Put the kettle on
Place pasta in the pot and bring to a boil (3 minutes)
Chop the salad vegetables and put them in a bowl
Drain the pasta

Serve... add grated cheese at the table.

14. SHEPHERD'S PIE

Time: Fridge to table: 1 hour
   Effort: 30 minutes (although less if using mash from the previous day)

Ingredients
1 small bag of lamb mince
1 onion
1 clove garlic
1 tin chopped tomatoes
5 mushrooms
Tobasco/Worcester sauce/Teaspoon of chopped chilli (optional)
2 big potatoes per person for mash
Nob of butter and a splash of milk
Grated cheese
Frozen vegetables (beans, peas, broccoli, cauliflower)

Procedure
Put the oven on (190°C)
Put the kettle on
Chop the potatoes into small cubes and boil for 10 minutes
Chop the onion and shallow fry it with a splash of oil
Add garlic
Add mince (if frozen, that is fine)
Stir until the mince is brown
Add chilli, Tobasco, Worcester sauce, tomatoes and sliced mushrooms
Place on the lid and cook on low heat for 20 minutes
Drain the potatoes, add a nob of butter and a splash of milk and mash
Place the mince in a deep, large dish
Spoon mashed potatoes on top
Sprinkle grated cheese on top
Place in the oven for 30 minutes
Heat vegetables in the microwave (8 minutes).

Serve...

15. FISH PIE

Time: Fridge to table: 1 hour
Effort: 30 minutes (feels a bit frantic, although less if using mash from the previous day)

Ingredients
Fish mix:
2 pots of fish pie mix
1 onion

White sauce:
100 g butter
4 desert spoons of brown flour
1/2 pint of milk

Mashed potato:
2 big potatoes per person
Nob of butter
Splash of milk
Grated cheese

Procedure
Put the oven on (190°C)
Put the kettle on
Chop potatoes into cubes and boil for 10 minutes

Fish mix:
Chop the onion and shallow fry until soft
Add the fish pie mix (if frozen, that is fine)
Stir until cooking, then add the lid and cook for 20 minutes

White sauce:
Melt 100 g butter in a saucepan
Add the flour, stir and mix up.
Take off the heat and slowly add the milk
Bring back to the boil

Mashed potatoes:
Drain the potatoes
Add a nob of butter and a splash of milk
Mash up

Putting it together
Add the fish mix to a deep, large oven dish
Add white sauce on top
Spoon the mash on next
Run for over the top, then sprinkle on grated cheese.
Cook in the oven for 30 minutes
Heat vegetables in the microwave.

Serve ....

14. MEALS FOR WHEN YOU HAVE HAD ENOUGH

Sometimes, it all just seems like too much effort! So, here are some quick meals to keep your sanity. My motto is to aim high, so you have further to fall when you cannot manage it anymore. So, cook these meals now and again, but try to keep them as reserves rather than the mainstay of the family meals. And when you do cook them, you can still make them OK by always adding vegetables or salad.

- Fish fingers, chips (or potato wedges) and frozen vegetables
- Jacket potatoes, cheese and beans with frozen vegetables
- Help yourself to tea – brown bread, cheese, ham, hummus, salad (Peppers, cucumber, olives, chopped carrots, lettuce, tomatoes), leftovers
- Pizza with salad and garlic bread
- Burgers, potato wedges and salad
- Chicken kievs, potato wedges and frozen vegetables
- Fish and chips and peas

RESOURCES AND CONNECTIONS

Here are some books and websites that you might find useful:

BOOKS

Bryant-Waugh, R., and Lask, B. (2013). *Eating Disorders: A Parents' Guide,* 2nd ed. London: Routledge.

Hunt, C., and Mountford, A. (2003). The parenting puzzle. The family links Nurturing Programme. Family links.

Ogden, J. (2014). The good parenting food guide: Managing what children eat without making food a problem. Wiley Blackwell: Oxford. Made Open Access (2021).

Ogden, J. (2018). *The Psychology of Dieting.* London: Routledge.

Treasure, J., and Alexander, J. (2013). *Anorexia Nervosa: A Recovery Guide for Sufferers, Families and Friends.* London: Routledge.

ARTICLES FOR THE GENERAL PUBLIC

Here are some articles I have written for the general public that you might find interesting:

Ogden, J. (2013). Banning packed lunches is a step too far. *The Conversation.* https://theconversation.com/banning-packed-lunches-is-a-step-too-far-16155

Ogden, J. (2013). Jamie's right: Ready meals are a modern curse. *The Conversation.* http://theconversation.com/jamies-right-ready-meals-are-a-modern-curse-17669

Ogden, J. (2013). Nick Clegg is spot on over free school meals. *The Conversation.* http://theconversation.com/nick-clegg-is-spot-on-over-free-school-meals-18375

Ogden, J. (2013). Sugar hysteria won't solve the obesity problem. *The Conversation*. http://theconversation.com/sugar-hysteria-wont-solve-the-obesity-puzzle-17384

Ogden J. (2014). Attacks on nanny state are propped up by vested interests. The Conversation. https://theconversation.com/columns/jane-ogden-96406

Ogden, J. (2014). Free obesity surgery on the NHS is worth the money. The Conversation. http://theconversation.com/free-obesity-surgery-on-the-nhs-is-worth-the-money-34818

Ogden, J. (2014). Let's put the 'school' back into free school meals and teach our children the importance of good diet. The Conversation. https://theconversation.com/lets-put-the-school-back-into-free-school-meals-and-teach-the-importance-of-good-diet-31124

Ogden, J. (2014). Obesity by any other name would still be fat. *The Conversation* https://theconversation.com/obesity-by-any-other-name-would-still-be-fat-22600

Ogden, J. (2014). Obesity is now so normal that many parents can't see if their child is too fat. *The Conversation*. https://theconversation.com/obesity-is-now-so-normal-that-many-parents-cant-see-if-their-child-is-too-fat-31032

Ogden, J. (2014). The no headline headline: Just eat less and do more. *The Huffington Post*. www.huffingtonpost.co.uk/jane-ogden/the-no-headline-headline-just-eat-less-and-do-more_b_5882496.html

Ogden, J. (2015). Are we normalising obesity? *The independent online*. http://www.independent.co.uk/life-style/health-and-families/features/are-we-normalising-obesity-10313776.html

Ogden, J. (2015). Cap sugar fat and salt. *The Conversation*. http://theconversation.com/cap-sugar-fat-and-salt-three-hours-of-exercise-a-day-labours-plan-for-unhealthy-kids-36309

Ogden, J. (2015). Eight sneaky tips to encourage your children to eat healthy foods. *The Conversation*. https://theconversation.com/eight-sneaky-tricks-to-get-your-children-to-eat-healthy-food-39284

Ogden, J. (2015). How much sugar is lurking in your cereal? *The Conversation*. http://theconversation.com/how-much-sugar-is-lurking-in-your-cereal-36797

Ogden, J. (2015). Thank you bikini terrorists for moving us on from throwback diet ads. *The Conversation*. https://theconversation.com/thank-you-bikini-terrorists-for-moving-us-on-from-throwback-diet-ads-now-eachbodysready-40973

Ogden, J. (2016). Eating well – its more than just what you eat. *The Conversation*. https://theconversation.com/eating-well-its-more-than-just-what-you-eat-52916

Ogden, J. (2016). Jamie Oliver's big chance to persuade the world to take action against obesity. *The Conversation*. http://theconversation.com/jamie-olivers-big-chance-to-persuade-the-world-to-take-action-against-obesity-59833#comment_983928

Ogden, J. (2016). Now we can't walk if we want to. *International Business Times*. www.ibtimes.co.uk/now-we-cant-walk-if-we-want-tfls-nanny-state-lesson-laziness-1549676.

Ogden, J. (2016). Ten mind tricks to make you a healthier eater. *The Daily Mail*. www.thisismoney.co.uk/health/article-3448464/Ten-mind-tricks-make-healthier-eater.html?hootPostID=cfeef6ee6c29e38df12cd46838c1e796

Ogden, J. (2016). When it comes to food its not helpful to believe in the genetics of behaviour. *The Conversation*. https://theconversation.com/when-it-comes-to-food-its-not-helpful-to-believe-in-the-genetics-of-behaviour-67181

Ogden, J. (2017). Food labelled snack leaves your hungrier than food labelled meal. https://theconversation.com/food-labelled-snack-leaves-you-hungrier-than-food-labelled-meal-86507.

Ogden, J. (2018). Don't dare tell us we're too old for bikinis. *The Daily Mail*. www.dailymail.co.uk/femail/article-5893125/Women-40-feel-confident-bikinis-20s.html

Ogden, J. (2020). Be kind to your body on lockdown and look to the diversity of people in the real world. https://theconversation.com/be-kind-to-your-body-on-lockdown-look-to-the-diversity-of-people-in-the-real-world-134089

Ogden, J. (2021). Preparing your own food or watching it being made could lead to overeating: New research. https://theconversation.com/preparing-your-own-food-or-watching-it-being-made-could-lead-to-overeating-new-research-154893

Ogden, J. (2022). The Sun. How to overcome overeating. www.thesun.co.uk/health/18461188/types-of-overeating-how-to-overcome/

Ogden, J. (2024). The i. I wish I'd told my children they were beautiful. https://inews.co.uk/inews-lifestyle/psychologist-wish-told-children-beautiful-2941099 March

Ogden, J. (2024). The words we use give our children scripts for life. Psychology Today.

Ogden, J. (2024). What lessons would we give to our younger selves. What Lessons Would We Give to Our Younger Selves? | Psychology Today.

Ogden, J. (2025). I'm a psychologist – seven ways to help your children to a healthier weight i news February.

Ogden, J. (2025). Why patients aren't always right. Psychology Today.

USEFUL WEBSITES

BEAT: The Charity for Eating Disorders offering advice and support. www.b-eat. co.uk/

Eating well in later life. www.malnutritiontaskforce.org.uk/sites/default/files/ inline-files/Eating%20well%20in%20later%20life%20-%20Final%20Ve rsion_2.pdf

Eating, drinking and ageing well – a new BDA resource for older people. www. bda.uk.com/resource/eating-drinking-and-ageing-well-a-new-bda-resou rce-for-older-people.html

Mumsnet: By parents for parents. www.mumsnet.com/

The NCT online support group. www.nct.org.uk/

For Product Safety Concerns and Information please contact our EU
representative GPSR@taylorandfrancis.com
Taylor & Francis Verlag GmbH, Kaufingerstraße 24, 80331 München, Germany

www.ingramcontent.com/pod-product-compliance
Lightning Source LLC
Chambersburg PA
CBHW061723270326
41928CB00011B/2089

```
* 9 7 8 1 0 3 2 9 8 7 2 5 5 *
```